Reduced rates
for members of immunological societies

AF887556

International Archives of Allergy and Immunology

Check the advantages of a subscription to International Archives of Allergy and Immunology

- ✔ published monthly
- ✔ regular publishing of reviews, commentaries and opinions on controversial subjects
- ✔ fast and high-quality publication guaranteed
- ✔ peer-reviewed articles only
- ✔ online subscription available in addition to a print subscription

2002: Volumes 127, 128, 129
4 issues per volume

Subscription rates per year for members of immunological societies

Subscription + postage and handling
CHF 208.– + CHF 57.60 Europe
CHF 208.– + CHF 85.50 Overseas
EUR 149.– + EUR 41.40
USD 159.00 + USD 57.60
+ online subscription per volume:
CHF 39.– / EUR 28.– / USD 30.00

Institutional rates per volume

Subscription + postage and handling
CHF 963.– + CHF 24.– Europe
CHF 963.– + CHF 35.60 Overseas
EUR 688.– + EUR 17.20
USD 741.00 + USD 24.00
+ online subscription per volume:
CHF 58.– / EUR 42.– / USD 45.00

Airmail surcharge per volume:
CHF 25.20 / USD 21.00

Prices subject to change
EUR price for Germany,
USD price for USA only

Society members receive 3 volumes (12 issues) for only

CHF 208.– / EUR 149.– / USD 159.00
(+ postage and handling)

For more information and a free online sample copy please log on to **www.karger.com/iaa**

KARGER

Order Form

International Archives of Allergy and Immunology

☐ **Please enter my 2002 subscription to International Archives of Allergy and Immunology:**

☐ Members of immunological societies (rates per year):
CHF 208.– + CHF 57.60 Europe
CHF 208.– + CHF 85.50 Overseas
EUR 149.– + EUR 41.40
USD 159.00 + USD 57.60

☐ I am a member of the following society:

____

☐ Institutional

Chemical Immunology

Please send __ copy/ies of volume____
ISBN 3–8055–

☐ Institutions ☐ Individuals

☐ information on previous volumes

☐ information on publications in related fields

Payment:

☐ Check enclosed
☐ Please bill me
☐ Credit card
☐ American Express ☐ Visa ☐ Diners
☐ MasterCard ☐ Eurocard

Card No.: ______________________

Exp. date: ______________________

Name/Address:

____

____

____

E-Mail: ______________________

Date/Signature:

____

KI 02219

Chemical Immunology

'... There can be few immunologists in a position to ignore the help provided by these timely reviews ... essential reading for virtually all immunologists.' *Immunology*

Series Editors: **Adorini, L.** *(Milan);* **Arai, K.** *(Tokyo);* **Berek, C.** *(Berlin);* **Schmitt-Verhulst, A.-M.** *(Marseille);* **Waksman, B.H.** *(New York, N.Y.)*

Appearing for the first time in 1939, 'Progress in Allergy' was the first and, for many years, the only international review series in the English language devoted to immunology. The present title, 'Chemical Immunology', reflects the rapidly increasing role of concepts and techniques of molecular and cell biology, as well as the greater emphasis now being placed on research into the biologic problems of im-munology, hypersensitivity and immunopathology. Highly specialized, single-topic volumes keep both investigators and practicing physicians up to date with the latest developments in areas of immunology where recent research has been concentrated.

KARGER

Please enquire about the special price for members of immunological societies

For more information on these and previous volumes, please log on to: **www.karger.com/bookseries/chemi**

place stamp here

International Archives of Allergy and Immunology

Chemical Immunology

S. Karger AG
P.O. Box
CH–4009 Basel
(Switzerland)

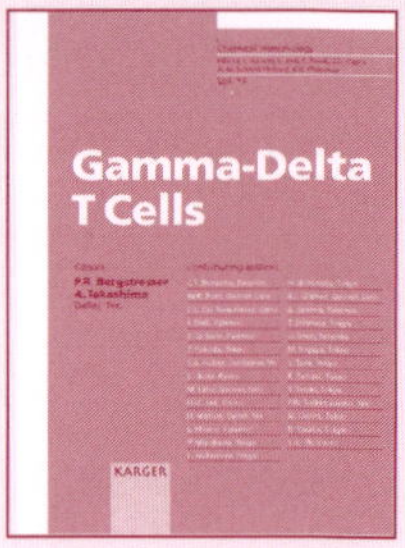

Vol. 79: Gamma-Delta T Cells
Editors: Bergstresser, Paul R.; Takashima, Akira (Dallas, Tex.)
X + 142 p., 23 fig., 9 tab., soft cover, 2001
Institutions: CHF 178.–/EUR 127.–/USD 15
Individuals: CHF 89.–/EUR 63.50/USD 77.5
ISBN 3–8055–7205–0

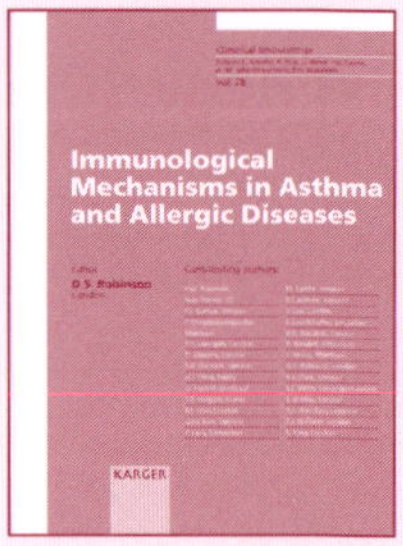

Vol. 78: Immunological Mechanisms in Asthma and Allergic Diseases
Editor: Robinson, D.S. (London)
XII + 214 p., 26 fig., hard cover, 2000
Institutions: CHF 256.–/EUR 183.–/USD 22
Individuals: CHF 128.–/EUR 91.50/USD 11
ISBN 3–8055–7112–7

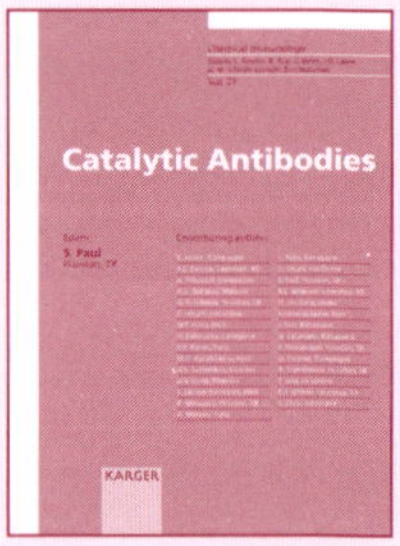

Vol. 77: Catalytic Antibodies
Editor: Paul, S. (Houston, Tex.)
X + 162 p., 58 fig., 3 in color, 10 tab., hard cover, 2000
Institutions: CHF 197.–/EUR 140.50/USD
Individuals: CHF 98.50/EUR 70.50/USD 85
ISBN 3–8055–7099–6

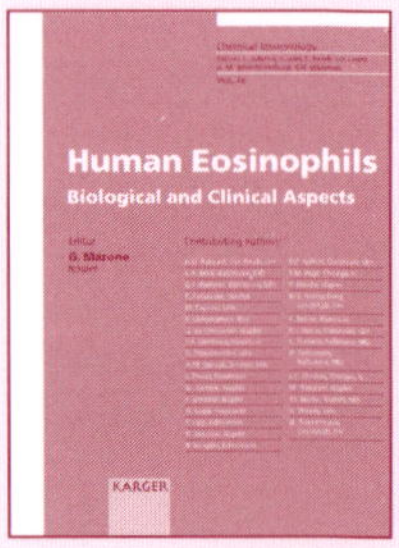

Vol. 76: Human Eosinophils
Biological and Clinical Aspects
Editor: Marone, G. (Naples)
XIV + 250 p., 47 fig., 13 in color, 17 tab., hard cover, 2000
Institutions: CHF 238.–/EUR 170.–/USD 2
Individuals: CHF 119.–/EUR 85.–/USD 103
ISBN 3–8055–6974–2

Prices subject to change
EUR price for Germany,
USD price for USA only

Official Journal of the Collegium Internationale Allergologicum

International Archives of Allergy and Immunology

Founded 1950 by D. Harley, P. Kallós, W. Löffler and F.W. Wittich
Continued by E.A. Brown (1952–1954), W. Kaufman (1955–1967),
F. Hahn (1961–1972), H.C. Goodman (1963–1975),
R.R.A. Coombs (1955–1984), Z. Trnka (1972–1987), P. Kallós (1950–1988),
G.B. West (1959–1991), J. Bienenstock (1990–1991), L.Å. Hanson (1981–1991),
K. Kano (1982–1991), F. Milgrom (1965–1991), K. Rother (1982–1991),
G. Wick (1991–1997), B. Grubeck-Loebenstein (1991–1997)

Editor-in-Chief

D. Kraft, Vienna

Managing Editor

R. Valenta, Vienna

Associate Editors

K. Blaser, Davos
M.D. Chapman, Charlottesville, Va.
K.T. HayGlass, Winnipeg
A.P. Kaplan, Charleston, S.C.
J. Lamb, Edinburgh
R. O'Hehir, Prahran, Melb.
R. Pawankar, Tokyo
A. Radbruch, Berlin
H. Renz, Marburg/Lahn
M. Röllinghof, Erlangen
H. Saito, Tokyo
W. Thomas, Perth
M. Triggiani, Naples
D. Vercelli, Tucson, Ariz.
R. Würzner, Innsbruck

Consulting Editor for Biostatistics
M. Kundi, Vienna

Editorial Board

G. Boltz-Nitulescu, Vienna
J. Bousquet, Montpellier
M. Breitenbach, Salzburg
H. Breiteneder, Vienna
A. Bufe, Bochum
A.W. Burks, Little Rock, Ark.
M. Capron, Lille
R. Crameri, Davos
C.A. Dahinden, Bern
S.R. Durham, London
A.M. Dvorak, Boston, Mass.
C. Ebner, Vienna
F. Ferreira, Salzburg
E.W. Gelfand, Denver, Colo.
P.G. Holt, Perth
D. Kabelitz, Kiel
A. Kapp, Hannover
M.L. Kapsenberg, Amsterdam
H. Lassmann, Vienna
S. Lehrer, New Orleans, La.
E. Maggi, Florence
R.N. Maini, London
F. Melchers, Basel
G. Opelz, Heidelberg
I. Pecht, Rehovot
W.J. Pichler, Bern
T.A.E. Platts-Mills, Charlottesville, Va.
R. van Ree, Amsterdam
H.-R. Rodewald, Ulm
L.J. Rosenwasser, Denver, Colo.
P. Rothman, New York, N.Y.
J.-M. Saint-Rémy, Leuven
H.A. Sampson, New York, N.Y.
O. Scheiner, Vienna
T. Schwarz, Münster
Y. Shoenfeld, Tel Hashomer
H.-U. Simon, Bern
J. Smolen, Vienna
B.M. Stadler, Bern
G. Stingl, Vienna
H. Stockinger, Vienna
P. Valent, Vienna
H. Wekerle, Martinsried
G. Wick, Innsbruck
H. Yssel, Montpellier

KARGER

Printed in Switzerland on acid-free paper by Reinhardt Druck, Basel

Appears monthly: 3 volumes per year (12 issues)

Guidelines for Authors

International Archives of
Allergy and
Immunology

'International Archives of Allergy and Immunology' appears monthly and provides a forum for publication of work from all aspects of modern allergology and immunology. Papers considered of special interest will be treated as 'hot topics' and every attempt will be made to publish these especially fast. Starting in 1998, a new Editor-in-Chief, Managing Editor and a team of internationally established Associate Editors competently covering all fields of allergology and immunology will be responsible for the scientific quality of this international core journal. *International Archives* will publish original work in the fields of allergy, immunopathology and transplantation, cellular immunology, immunogenetics, immunopharmacology and immunoendocrinology, mucosal immunity, immunology of infectious diseases and immunology of connective tissue diseases. In addition, reviews, minireviews, commentaries and opinions on controversial subjects will be published regularly. A new system of manuscript submission, reviewing and processing will guarantee competent and fair reviewing as well as fast and high quality publication.

Submission

Only papers written in English are considered. Manuscripts should be submitted in triplicate (with three sets of illustrations of which one is an original), typewritten double-spaced on one side of the paper, with a wide margin. The papers should be sent to:

Prof. Dr. D. Kraft
Editor-in-Chief
S. Karger AG
Editorial Office International Archives of
Allergy and Immunology
PO Box
CH–4009 Basel (Switzerland)
Tel. +41 61 306 1360
Fax +41 61 306 1434
E-Mail e.lieberherr@karger.ch

Mailing address for courier deliveries only:

Allschwilerstr. 10
CH–4055 Basel (Switzerland)

Original research papers: Submitted manuscripts should be fully documented reports of original research. They must describe significant and original observations to be critically evaluated and, if necessary, repeated.

Short communications: These manuscripts should not contain more than **2 printed pages (i.e. 5 manuscript pages)**, including an abstract, essential references and not more than 3 tables or figures. Such communications should represent complete, original studies and should be arranged in the same way as full-length manuscripts.

Case reports of general immunological interest can be submitted.

Review articles, minireviews and commentaries: Authors who wish to contribute a manuscript to one of these categories should contact the Editor-in-Chief. Minireviews should be focused, brief reports on topics of current interest. Commentaries should offer a more personalized perspective on a topic that will be of interest to the general readership. All contributions to these categories will be subject to Editorial review.

Letters to the Editor concerning work published in the journal may be submitted. They should not exceed 2 manuscript pages including one table or figure.

Conditions

All manuscripts are subject to editorial review. Manuscripts are received with the explicit understanding that they are not under simultaneous consideration by any other publication. A cover letter with the name, address, and telephone and telefax numbers of the corresponding author must accompany each manuscript. This letter must include a statement that affirms that all authors agree with the submission. Submission of an article for publication implies the transfer of the copyright from the author to the publisher upon acceptance. Accepted papers become the permanent property of 'International Archives of Allergy and Immunology' and may not be reproduced by any means, in whole or in part, without the written consent of the publisher. It is the author's responsibility to obtain permission to reproduce illustrations, tables, etc. from other publications. One of the criteria considered in reviewing manuscripts is the proper treatment of animals. In particular, the use of painful or otherwise noxious stimuli must be carefully and thoroughly justified. Papers that do not meet these criteria will not be accepted for publication.

Arrangement

Title page: The first page of each paper should indicate the title, the authors' names, and the institution where the work was conducted. A short title for use as running head is also required.

Key words: A list of 3–10 key words should be included for indexing purposes.

Abstract: **Provide on a separate page an abstract of not more than 250 words. This abstract should consist of four paragraphs, labeled Background, Methods, Results, and Conclusions. They should briefly describe, respectively, the problem being addressed in the study, how the study was performed, the salient results, and what the authors conclude from the results.**

The text should be arranged in the following sections: Introduction, Material and Methods, Results, Discussion, Acknowledgement, References.

Small type: Paragraphs which can or must be set in smaller type (case histories, test methods, etc.) should be indicated with a 'p' (petit) in the margin on the left-hand side.

Footnotes: Avoid footnotes. When essential, they are numbered consecutively and typed at the foot of the appropriate page.

Tables and illustrations: Tables and illustrations (both numbered in Arabic numerals) should be prepared on separate sheets. Tables require a heading and figures a legend, also prepared on a separate sheet. For the reproduction of illustrations, only good drawings and original photographs can be accepted; negatives or photocopies cannot be used. Due to technical reasons, figures with a screen background should not be submitted. When possible, group several illustrations on one block for reproduction (max. size 181 × 223 mm) or provide crop marks. On the back of each illustration, indicate its number, the author's name, and 'top' with a soft pencil.

Color illustrations: Up to 6 color illustrations per page can be integrated within the text at the reduced price of CHF 660.– / USD 545.00 per page. Color illustrations are reproduced at the author's expense.

Abbreviations: Avoid overuse of abbreviations. Introduce an abbreviation only when the same term occurs three or more times.

References: In the text identify references by Arabic numerals [in square brackets]. Material submitted for publication but not yet accepted should be noted as 'unpublished data' and not be included in the reference list. The list of references should include only those publications which are cited in the text. Do not alphabetize; number references in the order in which they are first mentioned in the text. The surnames of the authors followed by initials should be given. There should be no punctuation other than a comma to separate the authors. Cite all authors, 'et al' is not sufficient. Abbreviate journal names according to the Index Medicus system. (Also see International Committee of Medical Journal Editors: Uniform requirements for manuscripts submitted to biomedical journals. N Engl J Med 1997;336:309–315.)

Examples

(a) Papers published in periodicals: Sun J, Koto H, Chung KF: Interaction of ozone and allergen challenges on bronchial responsiveness and inflammation in sensitised guinea pigs. Int Arch Allergy Immunol 1997;112:191–195.

(b) Monographs: Matthews DE, Farewell VT: Using and Understanding Medical Statistics, ed 3, revised. Basel, Karger, 1996.

(c) Edited books: Parren PWHI, Burton DR: Antibodies against HIV-1 from phage display libraries: Mapping of an immune response and progress towards antiviral immunotherapy; in Capra JD (ed): Antibody Engineering. Chem Immunol. Basel, Karger, 1997, vol 65, pp 18–56.

Full address: The exact postal address complete with postal code must be given at the bottom of the title page. Please also supply phone and fax numbers, as well as your e-mail address.

Page charges

There are no page charges for papers of 5 or fewer printed pages (including tables, illustrations and references). Each additional complete or partial page is charged to the author at CHF 275.– / USD 196.–. The allotted size of a paper is equal to approx. 14 manuscript pages (including tables, illustrations and references).

Galley proofs

Unless indicated otherwise, galley proofs are sent to the first-named author and should be returned with the least possible delay. Alterations made in galley proofs, other than the correction of printer's errors, are charged to the author. No page proofs are supplied.

Reprints

Order forms and a price list are sent with the galley proofs. Orders submitted after the issue is printed are subject to considerably higher prices.

KARGER

Fax+ 41 61 306 12 34
E-Mail karger@karger.ch
www.karger.com

© 2002 S. Karger AG, Basel

The Guidelines for Authors are available at:
www.karger.com/journals/iaa/iaa_gl.htm

General Information

International Archives of
Allergy and
Immunology

Publication data: 'International Archives of Allergy and Immunology' is published 12 times a year. Volumes 127–129 with 4 issues each appear in 2002.

Subscription rates: Subscriptions run for a full calendar year. Prices are given per volume.

Personal subscription:
- *Subscription + postage and handling*
- CHF 481.50 + CHF 19.20 Europe
- CHF 481.50 + CHF 28.50 Overseas
- USD 370.50 + USD 19.20
- + online subscription per volume: CHF 39.– / USD 30.00
- (Must be in the name of, billed to, and paid by an individual. Order must be marked 'personal subscription'.)

Institutional subscription:
- *Subscription + postage and handling*
- CHF 963.– + CHF 24.– Europe
- CHF 963.– + CHF 35.60 Overseas
- USD 741.00 + USD 24.00
- + online subscription per volume: CHF 58.– / USD 45.00

Airmail postage: CHF 24.–, USD 20.00. (Extra per volume.)

Annual discount subscription prices:
- *Subscription + postage and handling*
- CHF 208.– + CHF 57.60 Europe
- CHF 208.– + CHF 85.50 Overseas
- USD 159.00 + USD 57.60

Members of following societies: AAAAI, AAI, BSACI, BSI, CSI, CIA, DGAI, DGI, EAACI, EFIS, ÖGAI, SFI, SGAI

Microforms: Please direct all enquiries and orders to: University Microfilms Inc.
300 North Zeeb Road, P.O. Box 1346
Ann Arbor, MI 48106-1346 (USA)

Subscription orders: Orders can be placed at agencies, bookstores, directly with the Publisher
S. Karger AG, P.O. Box
CH–4009 Basel (Switzerland)
or with any of the following distributors:
Deutschland: S. Karger GmbH, Postfach
D–79095 Freiburg
France: Librairie Luginbühl
36, bd de Latour-Maubourg, F–75007 Paris
Great Britain, Ireland: S. Karger AG
4 Rickett Street
London SW6 1RU, UK
USA: S. Karger Publishers, Inc.
26 West Avon Road, P.O. Box 529
Farmington, CT 06085, USA
India, Bangladesh, Sri Lanka:
Panther Publishers Private Ltd.
39, 6th Cross
Wilson Gardens
Bangalore 560 027, India
Japan: Katakura Libri, Inc.
2F, Marushima Bldg, 4-6-17 Yushima
Bunkyo-ku, Tokyo 113-0034, Japan

Change of address: Both old and new address should be sent to the subscription source.

Single issues and back volumes: Information can be obtained through the Publisher.

Advertising: Correspondence and rate requests should be addressed to the Publisher.

Bibliographic indices: This journal is regularly listed in bibliographic services, including *Current Contents®*.

Book Reviews: Books are accepted for review by special agreement.

Copying: This journal has been registered with the Copyright Clearance Center (CCC), as indicated by the code appearing on the first page of each article.
For readers in the US, this code signals consent for copying of articles for personal or internal use, or for the personal or internal use of specific clients, provided that the stated fee is paid per copy directly to
Copyright Clearance Center Inc.
222 Rosewood Drive
Danvers, MA 01923 (USA)
A copy of the first page of the article must accompany payment. Consent does not extend to copying for general distribution, for promotion, for creating new works, or for resale. In these cases, specific written permission must be obtained from the copyright owner,
S. Karger AG,
P.O. Box, CH–4009 Basel (Switzerland).

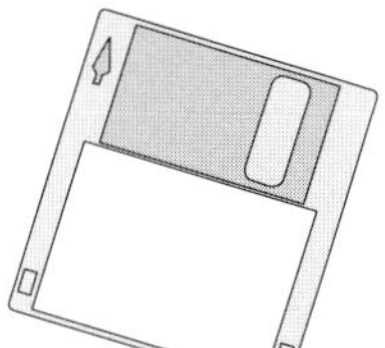

Disk Submission

A **comprehensive version** of these guidelines for the **submission of manuscripts and illustrations on disk** can be accessed online under **www.karger.com/journals/disksub.htm** or requested as a leaflet from the editorial department.

Please follow the general rules on style and arrangement in the **'Guidelines for Authors'** of the journal. Submit a **double-spaced printout** of your manuscript matching the file on disk exactly.

Technical Information

Store only data pertinent to this manuscript. Include your fonts (screen and printer fonts for Macintosh). For a **text only** manuscript, use a 3.5-inch disk. For **text and illustrations,** use 3.5 or 5.25 Magneto Optical Disc; CD-ROM (DOS or hybrid); iomage Zip/DOS (100 MB), or 44 MB, 88 MB or 200 MB SyQuest. Compress extensive data using ZIP format.

Data Description

Label your disk with the **title of the journal or book** for which it is submitted; a **short version** of the paper's title; your **name,** postal and e-mail address, fax and phone number; **hard- and software** used, including the version; and the **complete list of the file names.** File names consist of eight characters before the dot identifying the file and three characters after the dot identifying the application.

Text and Format

The **preferred word-processing package is MS-Word.** Other commonly used PC text programs and ASCII formats are accepted.
Update your data when you revise subsequent to the reviewer's or editor's decision and mark revisions clearly. Manuscripts accepted for publication are subject to **copy editing:** changes and/or questions will be marked in the manuscript, which will be returned to you with your disk and the galley proofs for checking.
Enter your text continuously flush left. Do not use any layout functions. Do not split words at the end of a line. **Do not use indentations.** Use a blank line before and a hard return at the end of paragraphs.
Arrange headings flush left. Insert only **one space after punctuation marks.** Insert Greek letters, mathematical symbols etc. with your word-processing program. Use **boldface and italics** as well as sub- and superscript where appropriate.
Tables are part of the text and should be placed at the end of the text file. Separate the individual parts of a table by lines. Use the tabulator instead of spaces. Format operation data on one line in the same column. **Legends to illustrations are part of the text** and should also be listed at the end of the text file.

Illustrations

Store illustrations as separate files: do not integrate them in your text. Export **line drawings/vector graphics** as TIF, EPS or WMF format. Use Photoshop for processing and retouching **scanned halftone images.** Save the original scan and the processed version. Export **black and white or color images** as TIF or EPS format in their anticipated size in print. **For detailed information** on how to submit illustration data on disk please consult the leaflet or **www.karger.com/journals/disksub.htm.**

KARGER

© 2002 S. Karger AG, Basel

Fax + 41 61 306 12 34
E-Mail karger@karger.ch
www.karger.com

The Journal Home Page is available at:
www.karger.com/journals/iaa

Karger journals and book series in ...

...Immunology

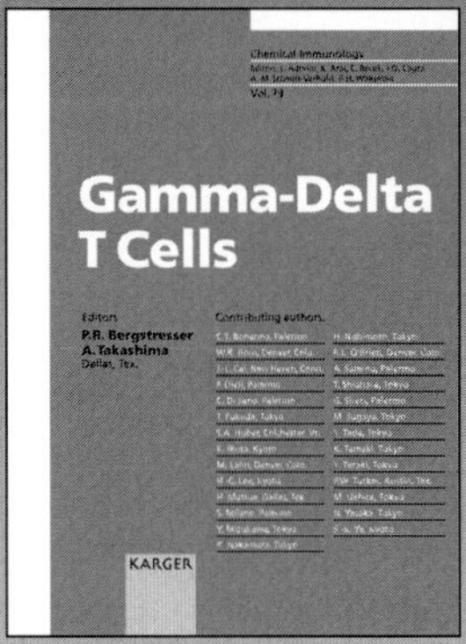

Chemical Immunology:
Highly specialized, single-topic volumes keep both investigators and practicing physicians up to date with the latest developments in all areas of immunology

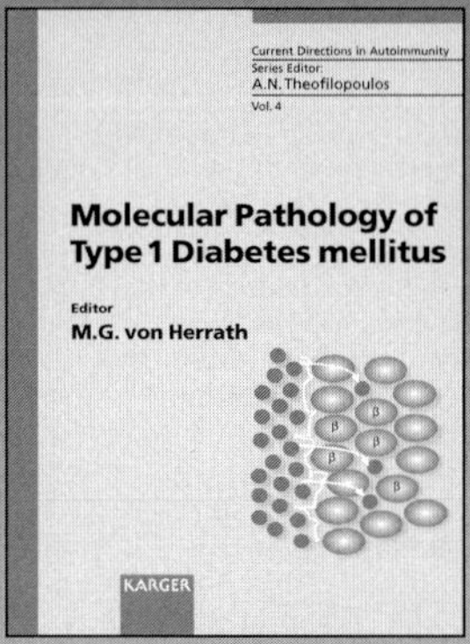

Current Directions in Autoimmunity:
This book series is designed to synthesize and consolidate current directions in basic and clinical research on autoimmunity

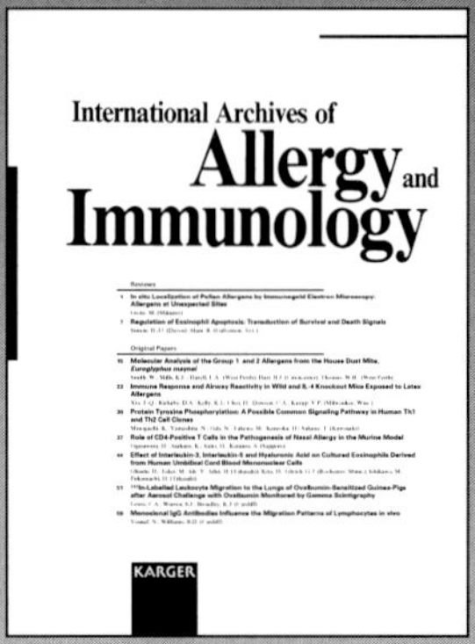

Established as a leading source of basic knowledge in all areas of modern molecular and cellular allergology and immunology

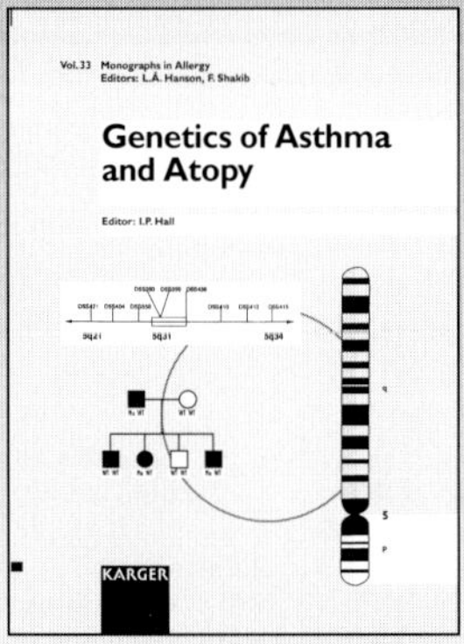

Monographs in Allergy:
Volumes in this series focus on areas of allergy and immunology characterized by exceptional importance and growth

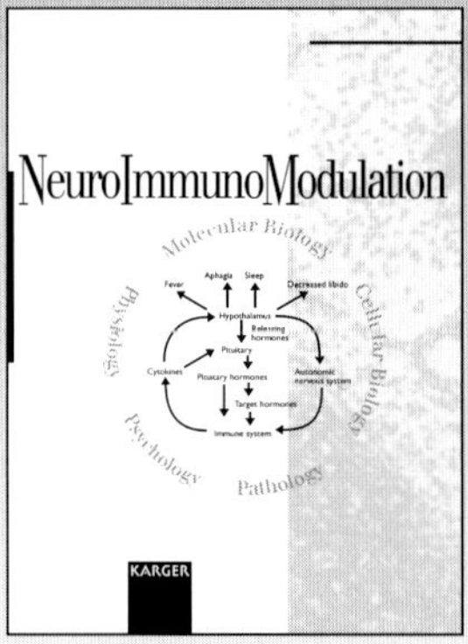

Encompassing both basic and clinical research, this journal investigates the complex interactions of the nervous and immune systems

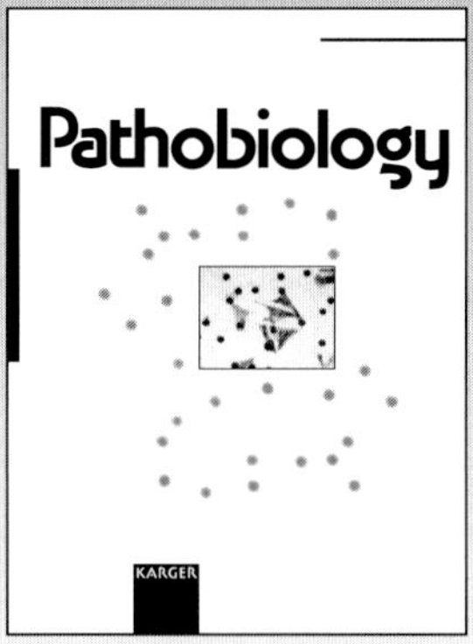

Original reports and interpretive reviews address timely topics in pathobiology, immunopathology, cellular and molecular biology, and medicine

Free journal sample copies available!

KARGER

S. Karger AG
P.O. Box, CH–4009 Basel
(Switzerland)
Tel. +41 61 306 11 11
Fax +41 61 306 12 34
E-mail karger@.karger.ch

S. Karger Publishers, Inc.
26 West Avon Road
P.O. Box 529
Farmington, CT 06085 (USA)
Toll free: 1-800-828-5479
Fax (860) 675-7302

For easy ordering or further information on Karger publications log on to:
www.karger.com

KI 02210

International Archives of
Allergy and Immunology

Eosinophils in Allergy and Related Diseases

Proceedings of a Workshop
Tokyo, Japan, June 16, 2001

Guest Editors
Sohei Makino, Tokyo
Takeru Ishikawa, Kumamoto
Takeshi Fukuda, Tochigi
Ken Ohta, Tokyo
Itsuo Iwamoto, Chiba
Takao Fujisawa, Mie

10 figures, 2002

KARGER
Basel · Freiburg · Paris · London · New York ·
New Delhi · Bangkok · Singapore · Tokyo · Sydney

S. Karger
Medical and Scientific Publishers
Basel · Freiburg · Paris · London
New York · New Delhi · Bangkok
Singapore · Tokyo · Sydney

Drug Dosage
The authors and the publisher have exerted every effort to ensure that drug selection and dosage set forth in this text are in accord with current recommendations and practice at the time of publication. However, in view of ongoing research, changes in government regulations, and the constant flow of information relating to drug therapy and drug reactions, the reader is urged to check the package insert for each drug for any change in indications and dosage and for added warnings and precautions. This is particularly important when the recommended agent is a new and/or infrequently employed drug.

All rights reserved.
No part of this publication may be translated into other languages, reproduced or utilized in any form or by any means, electronic or mechanical, including photocopying, recording, microcopying, or by any information storage and retrieval system, without permission in writing from the publisher or, in the case of photocopying, direct payment of a specified fee to the Copyright Clearance Center (see 'General Information').

© Copyright 2002 by S. Karger AG,
P.O. Box, CH–4009 Basel (Switzerland)
Printed in Switzerland on acid-free paper by
Reinhardt Druck, Basel
ISBN 3–8055–7447–9

KARGER

Fax + 41 61 306 12 34
E-Mail karger@karger.ch
www.karger.com

Vol. 128, Suppl. 1, 2002

International Archives of
Allergy and Immunology

Contents

KARGER

Fax + 41 61 306 12 34
E-Mail karger@karger.ch
www.karger.com

© 2002 S. Karger AG, Basel

Access to full text and tables of contents, including tentative ones for forthcoming issues:
www.karger.com/journals/ias/iaa_bk.htm

International Archives of
Allergy and
Immunology

Int Arch Allergy Immunol 2002;128(suppl 1):1–2

Preface

Takao Fujisawa

Mie, Japan

Allergic inflammation, as in bronchial asthma, is characterized by preferential recruitment of eosinophils into tissues. Increase in eosinophil numbers and/or their mediator concentrations in peripheral blood and tissues often correlate with disease activity, clinical severity, airway hyperresponsiveness, and airflow obstruction. A decrease in these concentrations with effective treatment is accompanied with improvement in symptoms and various physiological parameters such as lung function and airway responsiveness. Furthermore, studies on eosinophil biology over the last two decades have provided significant evidence that eosinophils are capable of causing inflammatory changes in allergic diseases. Thus, the 'eosinophil hypothesis' stating that eosinophils are the major effector cells in allergy has been proposed. However, a recent clinical trial in asthma with an anti-IL-5 monoclonal antibody has questioned the importance of eosinophils in allergic diseases including asthma [1], and has initiated a debate that has shaken the hypothesis and even societies of eosinophil research.

Leckie et al. [1] treated asthmatic patients with a humanized anti-IL-5 monoclonal antibody (SB-240563) to target eosinophils and found that allergen-induced late asthmatic responses (LAR) and nonspecific airway responsiveness did not change although the numbers of eosinophils in peripheral blood and sputum dramatically decreased. These findings argued against a central role of eosinophils in the pathogenesis of asthma. Logical criticism of the view that discounts the role of eosinophils based on initial clinical experience, however, has also emerged. First, LAR is not the right endpoint to evaluate eosinophil effector functions in asthma since basophils, not eosinophils, are directly involved in LAR [2]. Second, it was not clarified whether the antibody eliminated tissue eosinophils. If eosinophils remained in the tissue, they could still cause asthma. Actually, a subsequent study by Kay et al. [abstract presented at the 58th Annual Meeting of the American Academy of Allergy, Asthma, and Immunology, 2002] has found that SB240563 caused merely a 55% reduction of eosinophils in the lung although it caused an 88% reduction in peripheral blood. Furthermore, there is a report indicating that targeting IL-5 alone was not sufficient to block eosinophil infiltration in the lung and airway hyperresponsiveness [3]. Downregulation of IL-5 receptors and upregulation of GM-CSF receptors on tissue eosinophils in allergen-challenged asthmatics have also been suggested [Kelly, Busse, et al., pers. commun.]. Collectively, failure of the anti-IL-5 treatment does not necessarily minimize the pathogenic role of eosinophils. More studies will clarify whether targeting eosinophils will be useful in the treatment of asthma and whether IL-5 will be the effective target to treat eosinophilic inflammation.

In the midst of the heated debate on the role of eosinophils in asthma, the 14th Annual Workshop on 'Eosinophils in Allergy and Related Diseases 2001' was held in Tokyo on June 16, 2001, with 25 research presentations in the fields of basic and clinical sciences on eosinophil biology and its clinical correlations. Forefront researchers in this field in Japan presented and discussed their cutting-edge data including gene expression of eosinophils, the role of lipid mediators, cytokines, chemokines and adhesion molecules in eosinophil activation and mobilization, and the role of eosinophils in diseases with eosino-

KARGER

Fax + 41 61 306 12 34
E-Mail karger@karger.ch
www.karger.com

© 2002 S. Karger AG, Basel
1018–2438/02/1285–0001$18.50/0

Accessible online at:
www.karger.com/journals/iaa

philia. The effect of viral infection on eosinophilic inflammation was also discussed.

The present proceedings include two original papers and two reviews. Ten abstracts, some of which have been published elsewhere, are also included. The remaining eleven titles presented at the workshop are listed in the back of this issue. We hope that these studies will contribute to a better understanding and repositioning of eosinophils in allergy and eosinophil-related diseases.

Finally, we would like to express our sincere appreciation to Novartis Pharma K.K. (Tokyo) for supporting this workshop and to the International Medical Publisher (Tokyo) for excellent assistance in publishing these proceedings.

References

1 Leckie MJ, ten Brinke A, Khan J, Diamant Z, O'Connor BJ, Walls CM, et al: Effects of an interleukin-5 blocking monoclonal antibody on eosinophils, airway hyper-responsiveness, and the late asthmatic response. Lancet 2000;356:2144–2148.
2 Gauvreau GM, Watson RM, O'Byrne PM: Kinetics of allergen-induced airway eosinophilic cytokine production and airway inflammation. Am J Respir Crit Care Med 1999;160:640–647.
3 Webb DC, McKenzie AN, Matthaei KI, Rothenberg ME, Foster PS: Distinct spatial requirement for eosinophil-induced airways hyperreactivity. Immunol Cell Biol 2001;79:165–169.

Original Paper

International Archives of Allergy and Immunology

Int Arch Allergy Immunol 2002;128(suppl 1):3–11

Effect of Extracellular Matrix Proteins on Platelet-Activating Factor-Induced Eosinophil Chemotaxis

Mamoru Yoshikawa[a,b] Kenji Matsumoto[a] Makoto Iida[b] Akira Akasawa[a] Hiroshi Moriyama[b] Hirohisa Saito[a]

[a]Department of Allergy and Immunology, National Center for Child Health and Development Research Institute, and [b]Department of Otorhinolaryngology, Jikei University School of Medicine, Tokyo, Japan

Key Words

Eosinophil · Extracellular matrix protein · Integrin · Chemotaxis · Interstitial migration

Abstract

Background: Eosinophils accumulate in tissues during various allergic inflammatory processes. Selective eosinophil recruitment is the result of orchestrated events involving cell adhesion molecules and chemoattractants. However, the exact mechanism of the regulation of integrin avidity during interstitial migration is poorly understood. ***Objective:*** The purpose of this study was to investigate whether extracellular matrix proteins might activate human eosinophil chemotaxis and, if so, to clarify the mechanism in terms of integrin avidity. ***Method:*** Eosinophils were purified from the peripheral blood of healthy donors. Eosinophil migration was measured using Boyden chambers with filter membranes coated with fibronectin (Fn), vitronectin (Vn), laminin (Ln), hyaluronic acid, collagen type IV, or bovine serum albumin (BSA) overnight. Platelet-activating factor (PAF) was introduced into the lower chamber of each well. Eosinophils were placed in the upper chamber after incubation with IL-5 for 15 min. The number of eosinophils that transmigrated into the lower chamber was calculated by measuring the eosinophil peroxidase activity. ***Results:*** Fn, Ln and BSA enhanced PAF-induced chemotaxis of eosinophils. Inhibition experiments using blocking monoclonal antibodies showed that in the early phase of chemotaxis, Fn and Ln facilitated eosinophil chemotaxis that was mediated by $\alpha4$ and $\alpha6$ integrins, respectively. In the late phase of chemotaxis, BSA, but not other matrix proteins, facilitated both chemokinesis and chemotaxis that was mediated by $\beta2$ integrin. ***Conclusion:*** Our data strongly suggest that during chemotaxis, matrix proteins might activate eosinophils via binding with integrins to facilitate PAF-induced chemotaxis, and that such a mechanism might participate in allergic inflammatory processes.

Copyright © 2002 S. Karger AG, Basel

Introduction

In the last several years, numerous novel leukocyte chemoattractant receptors and their ligands have been identified. In general, several leukocyte subtypes express

KARGER

Fax + 41 61 306 12 34
E-Mail karger@karger.ch
www.karger.com

© 2002 S. Karger AG, Basel
1018–2438/02/1285–0003$18.50/0

Accessible online at:
www.karger.com/journals/iaa

Correspondence to: Dr. Kenji Matsumoto
Department of Allergy and Immunology
National Center for Child Health and Development Research Institute
3-35-31 Taishidou, Setagaya-ku, Tokyo 154-8567 (Japan)
Tel. +81 3 3416 0181, Fax +81 3 3414 8879, E-Mail kmatsumoto@nch.go.jp

these receptors in overlapping patterns, and each leukocyte subtype itself expresses multiple chemoattractant receptors. Many tissues have been designed with unique road patterns (adhesion molecules) with street signs and trafficking signals (chemokines) to direct subsets of leukocytes by selective interactions mediated by adhesion ligands and chemokine receptors [1]. Leukocytes have the capacity to respond sequentially to chemoattractants, making possible a step-by-step navigation through complex chemoattractant fields [2].

In particular, accumulation of eosinophils is observed in a variety of human diseases, including asthma and allergic rhinitis, and is considered to play a key role in the pathogenesis of these conditions [3]. Several laboratories have studied the mechanisms of eosinophil transendothelial migration into tissues from the vasculature [4, 5]. In previous studies, adhesion assays of purified ligands showed differential regulation of β1 integrin and β2 integrin avidity in eosinophils. Stimulus-induced down-regulation of β1 integrin function occurs along with up-regulation of β2 integrin activity [6, 7]. In another study, CCR3-active chemokines facilitate migration of eosinophils by shifting usage away from β1 integrin towards β2 integrin [8]. On the other hand, once eosinophils enter the extravascular space, migration through the tissue seems to be dependent on their ability to bind to extracellular matrix (ECM) proteins. Eosinophil migration into tissues is the result of coordinated events involving adhesion and deadhesion. However, the actual implication of ECM proteins in eosinophil interstitial migration is not clearly understood. The exact mechanism of the regulation of integrin avidity is also poorly understood. In tissues, a number of ECM proteins, including fibronectin (Fn), laminin (Ln), vitronectin (Vn), and collagen (Co), construct a complex local milieu which surrounds leukocytes [6]. Recent evidence indicates that the selectivity and flexibility necessary to regulate cell traffic under homeostatic and inflammatory conditions are provided by a differential tissue distribution of chemokines and regulated expression of chemokine receptors on different leukocyte subsets [9–11]. Eosinophils constitutively express α4β1 (CD49d/CD29), and they bind to the CS-1 region of Fn by means of this receptor. Eosinophils also express α6β1 (CD49f/CD29), and they bind to Ln via this receptor [12–16]. All granulocytes, including eosinophils, share the β2 integrins such as leukocyte-function-associated antigen-1 (LFA-1, CD11a/CD18), Mac-1 (CD11b/CD18), and p150,95 (CD11c/CD18). In particular, Mac-1 binds to fibrinogen and denatured protein [17–19].

We hypothesize that the avidity of β1 integrin and β2 integrin in eosinophils is differentially regulated during interstitial migration. To test this hypothesis, we investigated whether ECM proteins might activate human eosinophil chemotaxis and tried to clarify the mechanism in terms of integrin avidity.

Materials and Methods

Reagents

Human plasma Fn and plasma Vn were purchased from Asahi Techno Glass (Tokyo, Japan). Human plasma Ln, hyaluronic acid (HA), Co type IV (Co IV) and platelet-activating factor (PAF) were purchased from Sigma (St. Louis, Mo., USA). Bovine serum albumin (BSA) was purchased from Wako (Osaka, Japan). Recombinant human IL-5 was purchased from R&D Systems (Minneapolis, Minn., USA).

Monoclonal Antibodies

Blocking mouse IgG1 monoclonal antibodies (mAbs) recognizing α4 (HP2/1) and α6 (4F10) integrins were purchased from Serotec (Oxford, UK), a blocking mouse IgG1 mAb recognizing β2 (7E4) integrin was purchased from Immunotech (Westbrook, Me., USA), and an irrelevant mouse IgG1 control antibody (MOPC 21) was purchased from Sigma (St. Louis, Mo., USA).

Isolation of Human Eosinophils

Eosinophils were purified from the peripheral blood of healthy donors by using density gradient centrifugation and negative selection with immunomagnetic beads, as previously described [20]. Purity and viability were determined by Diff-Quik staining (American Scientific Products, McGraw Park, Ill., USA) of cytocentrifuge preparations and by trypan blue dye exclusion and were consistently greater than 98 and 99%, respectively (n = 20). The eosinophils were suspended in Hanks' Balanced Salt Solution (HBSS) containing 0.1% BSA at a concentration of 4×10^5 cells/ml. For priming, the eosinophils were incubated with IL-5 (1 ng/ml) for 15 min at 37 °C, prior to assay.

Eosinophil Chemotaxis Assays

Eosinophil migration was measured by the Boyden chamber technique using a 96-well multiwell plate (Neuro Probe Inc., Bethesda, Md., USA) and a 10-μm-thick polyvinylpyrrolidone-free polycarbonate filter membrane with pores 5 μm in diameter (Nero Probe Inc.) [21]. Filter membranes were coated overnight at 4 °C with 20-ml aliquots of Fn, Ln, Vn, HA, Co IV or BSA diluted in PBS. The concentration of the ECM protein coating was 25 μg/ml except for BSA (10 mg/ml), because, first, previous studies demonstrated that concentrations of ≥10 μg/ml significantly influence adhesion of ECM proteins to membranes [7, 14, 22], and second, in our preliminary experiments, ≥2.5 μg/ml ECM protein continuously showed a significant effect (data not shown). The filter membrane was washed twice with PBS, prior to assay. PAF was introduced into each well of the 96-well multiwell plate. This plate was placed in the bottom compartment of the assay chamber and covered with a framed filter membrane. The top compartment was carefully put in place, and the wing nuts were tightened to prevent leaking. Then, a cell suspension con-

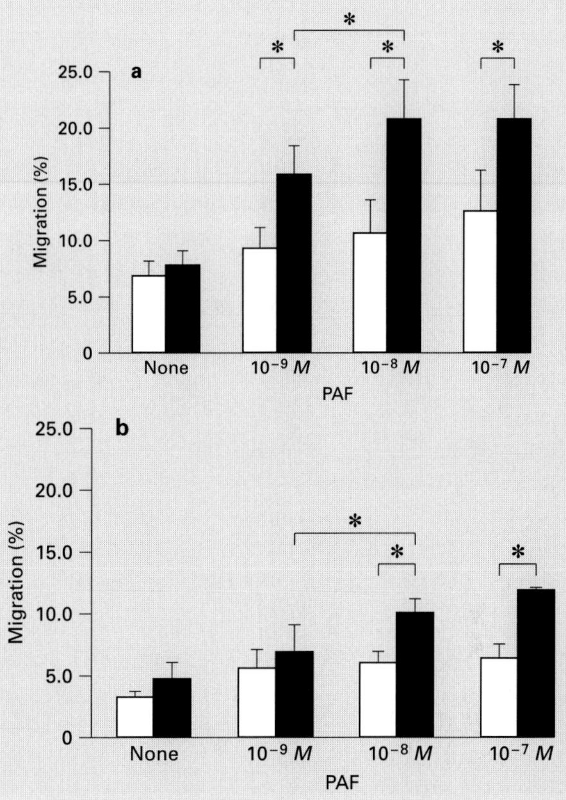

Fig. 1. Effect of Fn and Ln on PAF-induced chemotaxis. Polycarbonate filter membranes were coated overnight at 4 °C with 25 µg/ml Fn (**a**) or Ln (**b**). PAF was introduced into the lower wells (■) or not (□). The Boyden chamber was incubated for 60 min at 37 °C. Fn and Ln significantly facilitate PAF-induced eosinophil chemotaxis. Data are shown as the mean ± SEM of 4–7 separate experiments. * $p < 0.05$.

taining 4 × 10^4 purified eosinophils was introduced into the upper-compartment wells. In some experiments, a final mAb concentration of 10 µg/ml was added to the upper compartment wells simultaneously with the cell suspension and was allowed to remain throughout the chemotaxis assay. The chamber was incubated at 37 °C, in a 5% CO_2, humidified atmosphere.

Analysis of Migrated Eosinophils

After a certain time period, the wells of the upper compartment were emptied of fluid by aspiration, and the chamber was disassembled. To detach adherent eosinophils from the filter, the microtiter plate with its attached filter was placed on ice for 20 min and centrifuged at 400 *g* for 5 min at room temperature. The filter was carefully removed, and the supernatants were decanted by throwing. In this study, we used a rapid and sensitive eosinophil chemotactic assay system based on eosinophil peroxidase (EPO) determination [21]. The EPO activity was determined as previously described [23], with slight modification. In brief, 150 µl of 0.05 *M* Tris-HCl, pH 8.0, containing 0.1% (v/v) Triton X-100, 0.1 m*M* *o*-phenylenediamine dihydrochloride (OPD) (Sigma) and 1.0 m*M* hydrogen peroxide, was added to each well. The plate was left at room temperature to the desired extinction (usually within 10 min), and the reaction was terminated by addition of 50 µl of 4 *M* H_2SO_4. The optical density was measured at 490 nm in an ELISA reader (MR5000, Dynatech Laboratories Inc., Chantilly, Va., USA). Data were analyzed with the Biolinx 2.10 program (Dynatech Laboratories Inc.), and numbers of migrated eosinophils were calculated based on the calibration curve established with varying known numbers of eosinophils.

Statistical Analysis

Data are presented as the mean ± the standard error of the mean (SEM). Statistical significance was determined by the paired t test and considered significant at $p < 0.05$.

Results

Effect of ECM Proteins on PAF-Induced Eosinophil Chemotaxis

Coating the membrane with Fn or Ln significantly enhanced eosinophil chemotaxis induced by $\geq 10^{-9}$ *M* PAF or more than $\geq 10^{-8}$ *M* PAF, respectively (fig. 1).

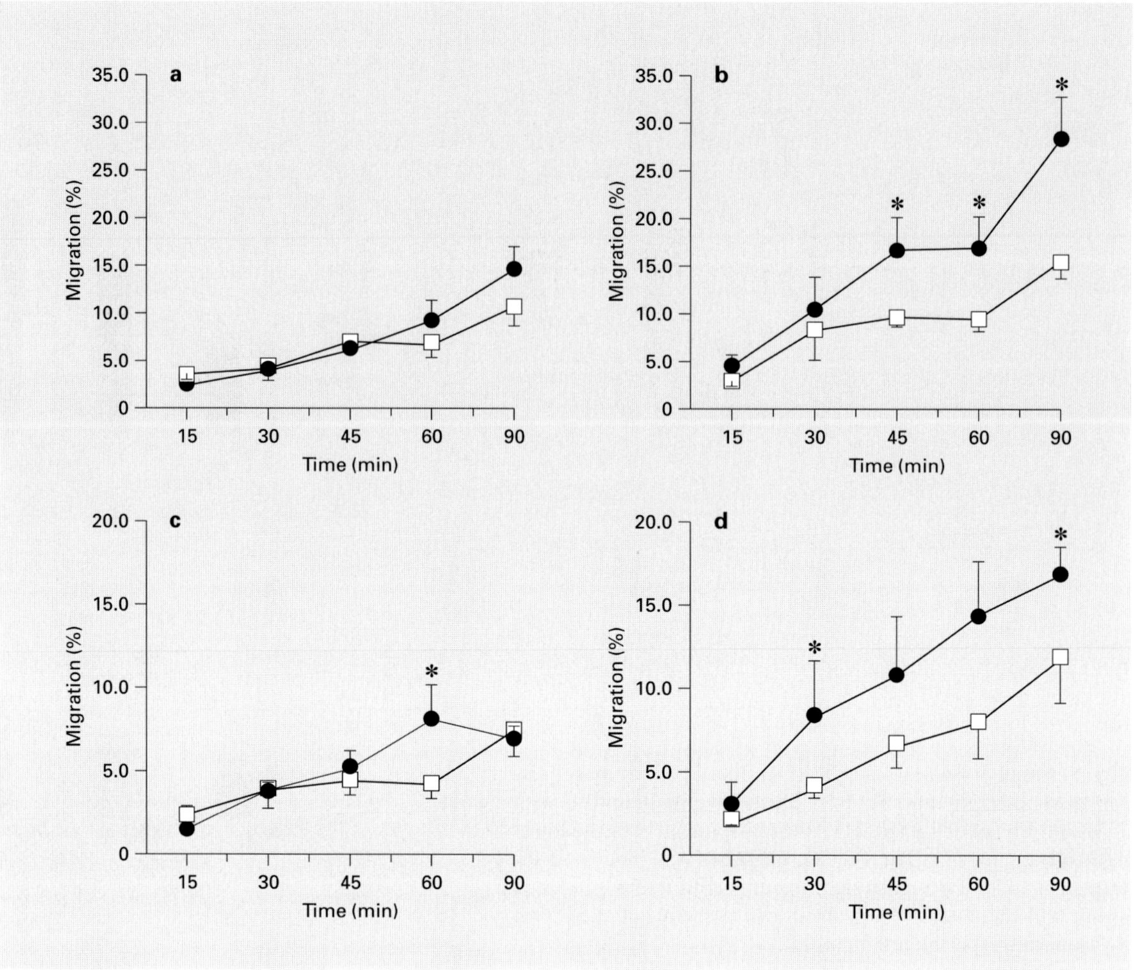

Fig. 2. Time kinetics of effect of Fn (**a**, **b**) and Ln (**c**, **d**) on PAF (10^{-8} *M*)-induced chemotaxis. Polycarbonate filter membranes were coated overnight at 4 °C with ECM protein (●) or without ECM protein (□) prior to the assay. The Boyden chambers were incubated at 37 °C. Migrated eosinophils were determined at various time points. Fn enhanced PAF-induced chemotaxis but not chemokinesis (**a**, **b**). Ln affected the PAF-induced chemotaxis and moderately affected chemokinesis (**c**, **d**). Data are shown as the mean ± SEM of 4–7 separate experiments. * $p < 0.05$.

Coating with Fn and Ln did not alter the chemokinesis of eosinophils. To determine when and how Fn and Ln affect eosinophil chemotaxis or chemokinesis, migrated cells were measured at various time points (15–90 min) (fig. 2). The percent migration of eosinophils was increased in a time-dependent fashion. In the presence of PAF, Fn and Ln enhanced PAF-induced chemotaxis of eosinophils. On the other hand, BSA enhanced both PAF-induced chemotaxis and IL-5-induced chemokinesis (fig. 3a). However, Co IV, HA and Vn had no effect on chemotaxis or chemokinesis (fig. 3b).

Effect of Integrin-Blocking mAb on PAF-Induced Eosinophil Chemotaxis

To examine which integrin participates in the activation of eosinophil chemotaxis by ECM proteins, inhibition assays were performed in the presence of blocking mAbs. Fn facilitated PAF-induced chemotaxis at 15 min that was abolished by α4 integrin-blocking mAb. It is noted that β2 integrin-blocking mAb showed no effect on PAF-induced chemotaxis. In contrast, chemotaxis at 60 min was almost completely inhibited by β2 integrin-blocking mAb, but not by α4-integrin-blocking mAb (fig. 4). The effect of Ln on PAF-induced chemotaxis was

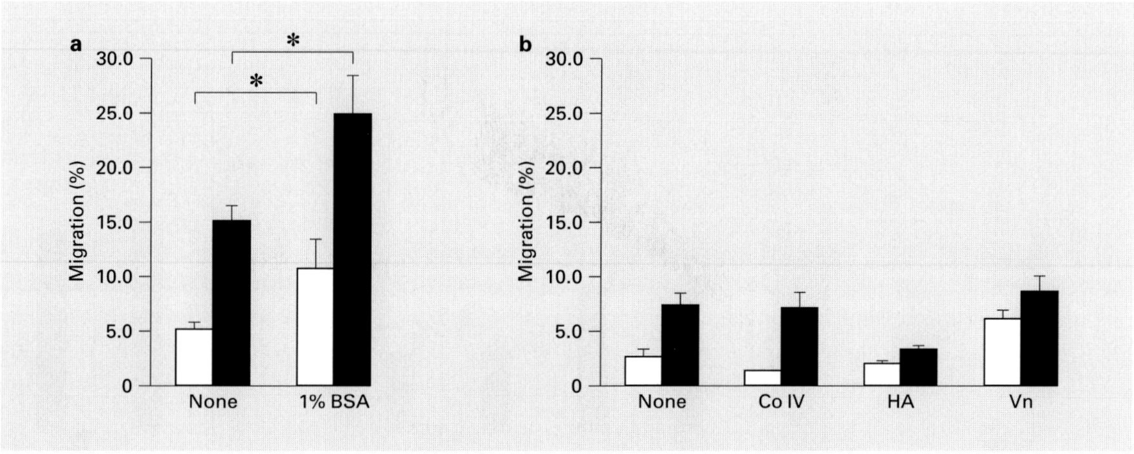

3

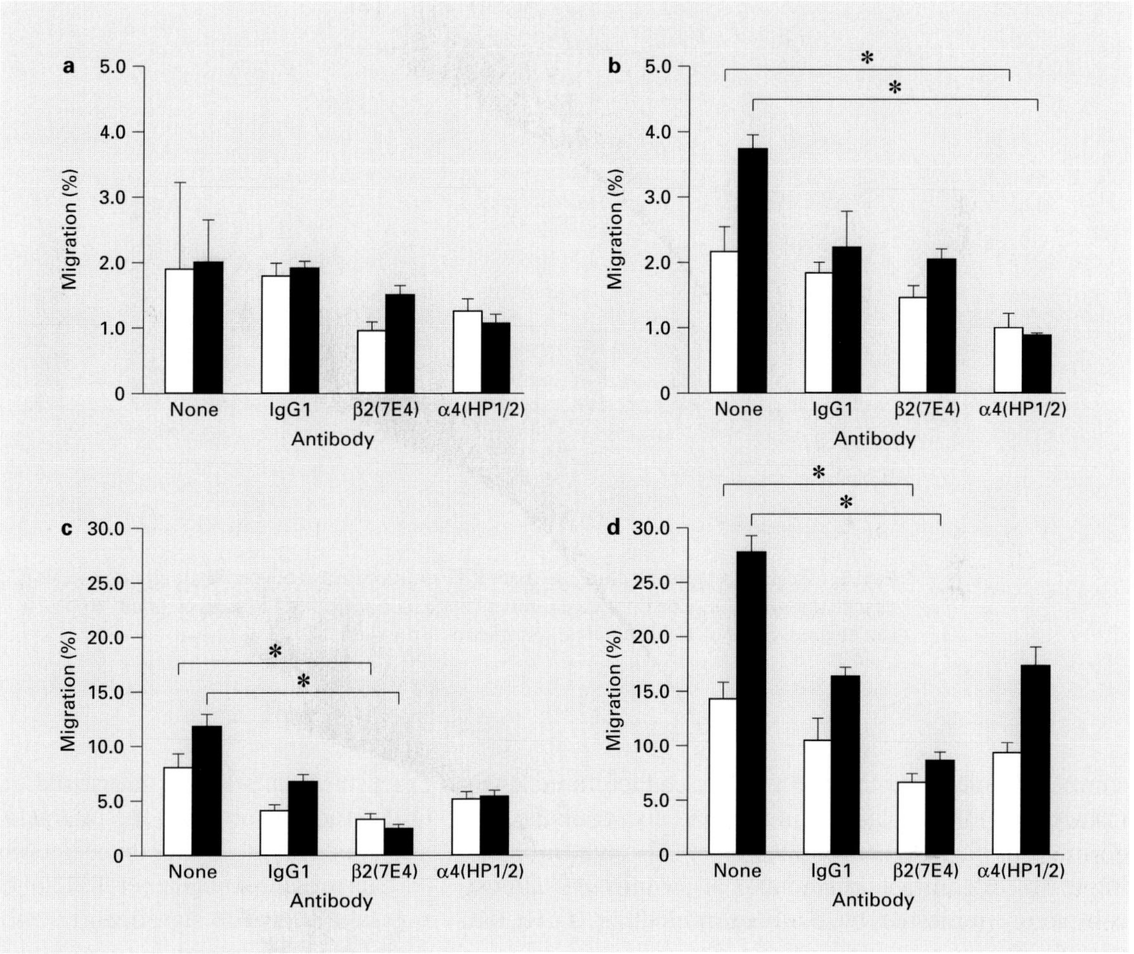

4

Fig. 3. Effects of other ECM proteins (**a, b**) on PAF-induced chemotaxis (■) or chemokinesis (□). Polycarbonate membrane filters were coated overnight at 4°C with or without ECM prior to assay. The Boyden chambers were incubated for 60 min at 37°C. BSA (**a**), but not Co IV, HA or Vn (**b**), significantly facilitated both PAF-induced chemotaxis and chemokinesis. Data are shown as the mean ± SEM of 3 separate experiments. * $p < 0.05$.

Fig. 4. Effect of integrin-blocking mAb on PAF-induced chemotaxis (■) or chemokinesis (□) in the presence (**b, d**) or absence (**a, c**) of Fn. The Boyden chambers were incubated for 15 (**a, b**) or 60 min (**c, d**) at 37°C. At 15 min of incubation, Fn enhanced PAF-induced chemotaxis that was almost completely abolished by mAb against α4 integrin. Data are shown as the mean ± SEM of 4–7 separate experiments. * $p < 0.05$.

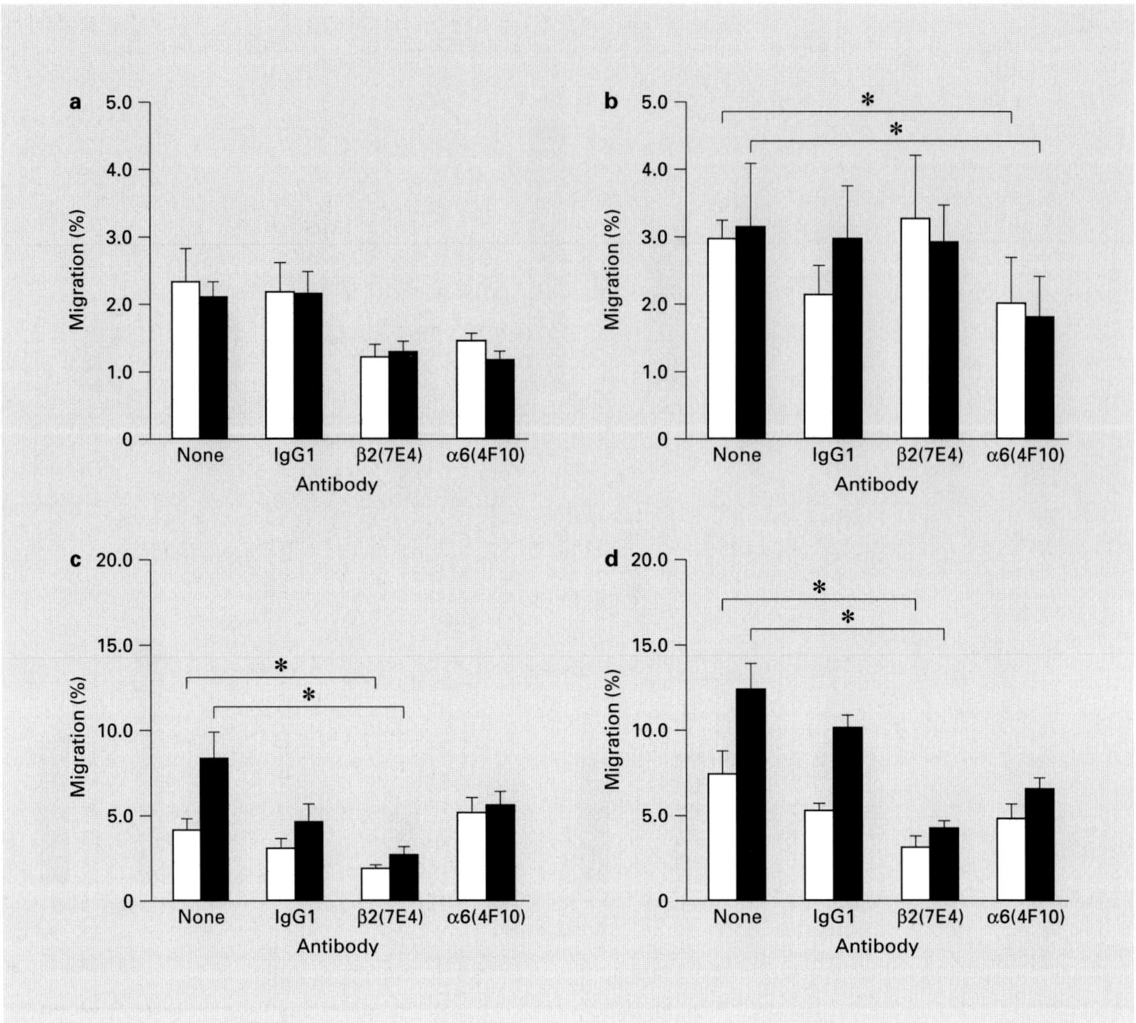

Fig. 5. Effect of integrin-blocking mAb on PAF-induced chemotaxis (■) or chemokinesis (□) in the presence (**b, d**) or absence (**a, c**) of Ln. The Boyden chambers were incubated for 15 (**a, b**) or 60 (**c, d**) min at 37 °C. Data are shown as the mean ± SEM of 4–7 separate experiments. * $p < 0.05$.

completely similar to the effect of Fn. Ln facilitated PAF-induced chemotaxis at 15 min that was also abolished by α6-integrin-blocking mAb, but not by β2-integrin-blocking mAb. In contrast, chemotaxis at 60 min was almost completely inhibited by β2-integrin-blocking mAb but not α6-integrin-blocking mAb (fig. 5).

Discussion

Recent studies have identified several mechanisms involved in the regulation of integrin avidity on eosinophils in transendothelial migration [6–8]. However, the exact mechanisms of interstitial migration are poorly understood. Especially, the interactions of ECM proteins and adhesion molecules on eosinophils remain unclear.

Our present study generated novel evidence that binding to Fn or Ln significantly enhances PAF-induced eosinophil chemotaxis but not chemokinesis. It was already reported that ameba-like movement of cells during chemotaxis is mediated by integrins on pseudopods [7]. Our present finding suggests that signaling through integrin selectively activates chemotactic movement of eosinophils, and that ECM proteins can act as handgrips for pseudopods for moving across a filter membrane.

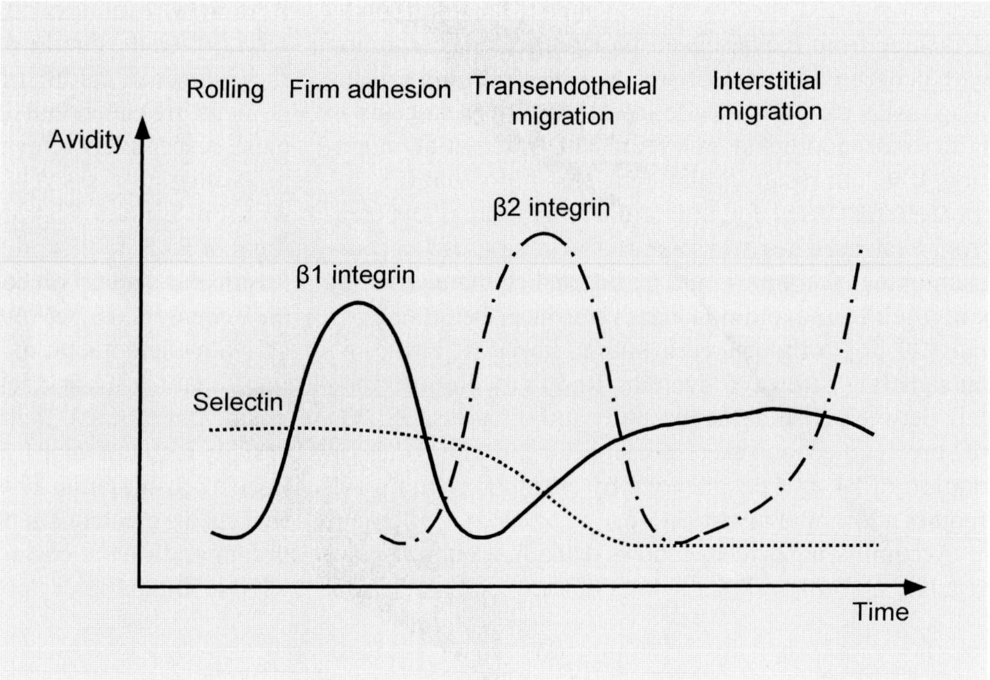

Fig. 6. Schema of avidity changes in adhesion molecules on eosinophils which might occur during recruitment into tissues. The horizontal axis indicates the time course, while the vertical axis indicates the avidity.

In addition, we also demonstrated that binding to Fn or Ln predominantly facilitates the early phase of PAF-induced chemotaxis. According to the blocking assays, that effect was mediated not by β2 integrin but by α4 and α6 integrins. In the late phase of chemotaxis, BSA but not the other ECM proteins facilitated PAF-induced chemotaxis, and that was mediated by β2 integrin.

During transendothelial migration of eosinophils, chemokines act through CCR3 to enhance the avidity of both α4 and β2 integrins reciprocally, thereby causing rapid eosinophil arrest under physiological conditions and enhancing LFA-1 affinity [24–27]. Our results strongly suggest that the avidity of α4, α6 and β2 integrins seems to be regulated in a fashion similar to transendothelial migration of eosinophils, and that shifting usage away from β1 integrin toward β2 integrin also occurs during interstitial migration.

Avidity changes in adhesion molecules on eosinophils which are surmised to occur during their recruitment from blood vessels into tissue sites are schematically shown in figure 6. In the first step, selectins and their carbohydrate ligands allow rolling of eosinophils on the vascular endothelium, leading to exposure of chemokine receptors to their ligands displayed on the surface of endothelial cells [28]. The triggering chemokine receptor results in a rapid activation of integrins, leading to firm adhesion and initiating transendothelial migration. In firm adhesion, β1 integrin avidity for vascular adhesion molecule 1 (VCAM-1) is up-regulated by exposure to chemokines through subsecond α4 integrin clustering at the leukocyte-substrate contact zone, but not by avidity changes in α4 integrin [29]. During this process, a reciprocal avidity change from β1 integrin to β2 integrin is induced at least in part by chemokines [6–8]. In the second step, detachment from intercellular adhesion molecule-1 (ICAM-1) on the endothelium, thereby initiating interstitial migration, was clarified in our present study. Exposure to chemokines such as PAF as well as binding to tissue Fn or basement membrane Ln induces up-regulation of chemotactic movement. At the same time, this stimulus down-regulates β2 integrin avidity, thereby promoting detachment from ICAM-1. During approximately 15 min to 1 h after eosinophils stop rolling, reciprocal β1 integrin avidity declines and β2 integrin avidity up-regulation is induced, thereby starting interstitial migration by detaching from the basement membrane and interaction with denatured proteins in tissues. Consequently, shifting usage away from β1 integrin toward β2 integrin occurs in both transendothelial migration and interstitial migration. If so, our results indicate the possibility that the chemoattractant used for interstitial migration is different from that used for transendothelial migration, because chemokine receptors would be internalized after binding with their ligand and no longer transduce chemokine signals [30, 31]. Although recent studies implicate intracellular signaling pathways involving Rho in mediating cross-talk between chemokine receptors and integrins [32, 33], the precise mechanisms responsible for the reciprocal regulation of β1 and β2 integrins by chemoattractants will require additional investigation.

Accumulating evidence shows that adhesion molecules regulate not only cell trafficking but also cell activation. Binding with an integrin itself is capable of activating cellular functions. On the other hand, cell activation reflects the changes in avidity of adhesion molecules. These phenomena are called 'outside-in signals' and 'inside-out signals', respectively. Our results show that human eosinophils migrate massively across filter membranes coated with Fn, Ln and BSA in response to a chemotactic gradient of PAF. In this process, both 'outside-in signals' and 'inside-out signals' on eosinophils are involved in eosinophil chemotaxis. As 'outside-in signals', ECM proteins activate chemotactic movement of eosinophils via binding with integrins and act as handgrips for pseudopods. As 'inside-out signals', chemoattractants such as PAF differentially regulate the β1 and β2 integrin-mediated chemotaxis of eosinophils. Therefore, our data strongly suggest that such a mechanism plays an important role in interstitial migration of eosinophils and might participate in allergic inflammatory processes.

References

1 Bochner BS: Road signs guiding leukocytes along the inflammation superhighway. J Allergy Clin Immunol 2000;106:817–828.
2 Foxman EF, Campbell JJ, Butcher EC: Multistep navigation and the combinatorial control of leukocyte chemotaxis. J Biol Chem 1997; 139:1349–1360.
3 Bochner BS: Systemic activation of basophils and eosinophils: Markers and consequences. J Allergy Clin Immunol 2000;106:S292–S302.
4 Bochner BS: Schleimer RP: The role of adhesion molecules in human eosinophil and basophil recruitment. J Allergy Clin Immunol 1994; 94:427–438.
5 Ebisawa M, Yamada T, Bickel C, Klunk D, Schleimer RP: Eosinophil transendothelial migration induced by cytokines. III. Effect of the chemokine RANTES. J Immunol 1994;153: 2153–2160.
6 Weber C, Kitayama J, Springer TA: Differential regulation of β1 and β2 integrin avidity by chemoattractants in eosinophils. Proc Natl Acad Sci USA 1996;93:10939–10944.
7 Matsumoto K, Sterbinsky SA, Bickel CA, Zhou DFH, Kovach NL, Bochner BS: Regulation of α4 integrin-mediated adhesion of human eosinophils to fibronectin and vascular cell adhesion molecule-1. J Allergy Clin Immunol 1997; 99:648–656.
8 Tachimoto H, Burdick MM, Hudson SA, Kikuchi M, Konstantopoulos K, Bochner BS: CCR3-active chemokines promote rapid detachment of eosinophils from VCAM-1 in vitro. J Immunol 2000;165:2748–2754.
9 Murphy-Ullrich JE: The de-adhesive activity of matricellular proteins: Is intermediate cell adhesion an adaptive state? J Clin Invest 2001; 107:785–790.
10 Márquez G, Martínez AC: Chemokines: The times they are a-changin'. J Clin Invest 2001; 107:791–792.
11 Sallusto F, Mackay CR, Lanzavecchia A: The role of chemokine receptors in primary, effector, and memory immune responses. Annu Rev Immunol 2000;18:593–620.
12 Buck CA, Horwitz AF: Cell surface receptors for extracellular matrix molecules. Annu Rev Cell Biol 1987;3:179–205.
13 Neeley SP, Hamann KJ, Dowling TL, McAllister KT, White SR, Leff AR: Augmentation of stimulated eosinophil degranulation by VLA-4 (CD49d)-mediated adhesion to fibronectin. Am J Respir Cell Mol Biol 1994;11:206–213.
14 Georas SN, McIntyre BW, Ebisawa M, Bednarczyk JL, Sterbinsky SA, Schleimer RP, Bochner BS: Expression of a functional laminin receptor (alpha 6 beta 1, very late activation antigen-6) on human eosinophils. Blood 1993; 82:2872–2879.
15 Kitayama J, Ikeda S, Kumagai K, Saito H, Nagawa H: Alpha 6 beta 1 integrin (VLA-6) mediates leukocyte tether and arrest on laminin under physiological shear flow. Cell Immunol 2000;199:97–103.
16 Hemler ME: VLA proteins in the integrin family: Structures, functions, and their role on leukocytes. Annu Rev Immunol 1990;8:365–400.
17 Harris ES, McIntyre TM, Prescott SM, Zimmerman GA: The leukocyte integrins. J Biol Chem 2000;275:23409–23412.
18 Plow EF, Haas TA, Zhang L, Loftus J, Smith JW: Ligand binding to integrins. J Biol Chem 2000;275:21785–21788.
19 Forsyth CB, Solovjov DA, Ugarova TP, Plow EF: Integrin αMβ2-mediated cell migration to fibrinogen and recognition peptides. J Exp Med 2001;193:1123–1133.
20 Hansel TT, Proud JD, Pilling D: Purification of human eosinophils by negative selection using immunomagnetic beads. J Immunol Methods 1989;122:97–103.
21 Nagase H, Yamaguchi M, Jibiki S, Yamada H, Ohta K, Kawasaki H, Yoshie O, Yamamoto K, Morita Y, Hirai K: A rapid and simple photometric assay for quantification of eosinophil chemotaxis. Int Arch Allergy Immunol 2000; 122 (suppl 1):10–14.
22 Kita H, Horie S, Gleich GJ: Extracellular matrix proteins attenuate activation and degranulation of stimulated eosinophils. J Immunol 1996;156:1174–1181.
23 Strath M, Warren DJ, Sanderson CJ: Detection of eosinophils using an eosinophil peroxidase assay. Its use as an assay for eosinophil differentiation factors. J Immunol Methods 1985;83: 209–215.
24 Constantin G, Majeed M, Giagulli C, Piccio L, Kim JY, Butcher EC, Laudanna C: Chemokines trigger immediate β2 integrin affinity and mobility changes: Differential regulation and roles in lymphocyte arrest under flow. Immunity 2000;13:759–769.
25 Kitayama J, Mackay CR, Ponath PD, Springer TA: The C-C chemokine receptor CCR3 participates in stimulation of eosinophil arrest on inflammatory endothelium in shear flow. J Clin Invest 1998;101:2017–2024.

26 Shahabuddin S, Ponath P, Schleimer RP: Migration of eosinophils across endothelial cell monolayers: Interactions among IL-5, endothelial-activating cytokines, and C-C chemokines. J Immunol 2000;164:3847–3854.
27 Jia GQ, Gonzalo JA, Hidalgo A, Wanger D, Cybulsky M, Gutierrez R: Selective eosinophil transendothelial migration triggered by eotaxin via modulation of Mac-1/ICAM-1 and VLA-4/VICAM4. Int Immunol 1999;11:1–10.
28 Knol EF, Kansas GS, Tedder TF, Schleimer RP, Bochner BS: Human eosinophils use L-selectin to bind to endothelial cells under nonstatic conditions. J Allergy Clin Immunol 1993; 91:334.
29 Grabovsky V, Feigelson S, Chen C, Bleijs DA, Peled A, Cinamon G, Baleux F, Arenzana-Seisdedos, Lapidot T, van Kooyk Y, Lobb RR, Alon R: Subsecond induction of α4 integrin clustering by immobilized chemokines stimulates leukocyte tethering and rolling on endothelial vascular cell adhesion molecule 1 under flow conditions. J Exp Med 2000;192:495–505.
30 Zimmermann N, Conkright JJ, Rothenberg ME: CC chemokine receptor-3 undergoes prolonged ligand-induced internalization. J Biol Chem 1999;274:12611–12618.
31 El-Shazly A, Yamaguchi N, Masuyama K, Suda T, Ishikawa T: Novel association of the src family kinases, hck and c-fgr, with CCR3 receptor stimulation: A possible mechanism for eotaxin-induced human eosinophil chemotaxis. Biochem Biophys Res Commun 1999;264: 163–170.
32 Laudanna C, Campbell JJ, Butcher EC: Elevation of intracellular cAMP inhibits RhoA activation and integrin-dependent leukocyte adhesion induced by chemoattractants. J Biol Chem 1997;272:24141–24144.
33 Laudanna C, Campbell JJ, Butcher EC: Role of Rho in chemoattractant-activated leukocyte adhesion through integrins. Science 1996;271: 981.

Original Paper

International Archives of Allergy and Immunology

Int Arch Allergy Immunol 2002;128(suppl 1):12–17

Histamine and Serotonin Stimulate Eotaxin Production by a Human Lung Fibroblast Cell Line

Etsuro Sato[a, b] Masayuki Haniuda[a] Hiroki Numanami[a] Toshiki Ushiyama[a] Akihiro Tsukadaira[a] Shuji Takashi[a] Yoshio Okubo[a] Sekiya Koyama[a]

[a]Shinshu University School of Medicine, Matsumoto, [b]Shinmachi Hospital, Shinshushinmachi, Nagano, Japan

Key Words
Eotaxin · Histamine · Serotonin · Chemotaxis

Abstract
Histamine and serotonin are important inflammatory mediators in the pathophysiology of asthma, and asthmatic patients have higher plasma histamine and serotonin levels than nonasthmatic control subjects. Eotaxin, a potent eosinophil-specific chemotactic factor, is increased in the lower respiratory tract of allergic patients. Recently, lung fibroblasts have been reported to produce eotaxin and are suggested to be the major cellular source of eotaxin. We postulated that lung fibroblasts might release eotaxin in response to histamine or serotonin. To test this hypothesis, we evaluated the potential of histamine or serotonin to induce the release of eotaxin by the human fetal lung fibroblast cell line, HFL-1. HFL-1 released eotaxin in response to histamine and serotonin in a dose- and time-dependent manner ($p < 0.05$). Histamine or serotonin treatment of HFL-1 augmented the expression of eotaxin mRNA. Eosinophil chemotactic activity by HFL-1 supernatant fluids was inhibited by anti-human eotaxin-neutralizing antibody. These findings lead to the hypothesis that lung-fibroblast-derived eotaxin may in part be responsible for the eosinophil infiltration observed in allergic disease of the airways.

Copyright © 2002 S. Karger AG, Basel

Introduction

It has long been known that eosinophils are present in increased numbers in the airways and peripheral blood of patients with severe asthma and it is now clear that even patients with mild intermittent asthma recruit these cells to the airways [1]. Eosinophil trafficking is regulated by a wide variety of chemotactic factors [2, 3]. However, the precise mechanisms are less certain. Eotaxin is a C-C chemokine purified from the bronchoalveolar lavage fluid (BALF) of actively sensitized guinea pigs after aerosol allergen challenge [4]. Eotaxin couples with C-C chemokine receptor 3 expressed on eosinophils, thus causing a selective recruitment of eosinophils to the sites of inflammation [5, 6]. Eotaxin is expressed on bronchial epithelial cells, T lymphocytes, macrophages, eosinophils, and lung fibroblasts [7–10].

KARGER
Fax + 41 61 306 12 34
E-Mail karger@karger.ch
www.karger.com

© 2002 S. Karger AG, Basel
1018–2438/02/1285–0012$18.50/0

Accessible online at:
www.karger.com/journals/iaa

Correspondence to: Dr. Etsuro Sato
Department of Internal Medicine
Shinmachi Hospital
137 Kamijo Shinshushinmachi, Nagano 381-2404 (Japan)
Tel. +81 26 262 3111, Fax +81 26 262 3411

In a variety of inflammatory airway disorders including bronchial asthma, several mediators are released by inflammatory cells and these mediators are believed to play an important role in the inflammatory responses. Among these, histamine and serotonin are important chemical mediators in the initiation and development of antigen induced immediate asthmatic responses including airway smooth muscle contraction and microvascular leakage [11, 12]. It is also reported that subjects with perennial asthma and those experiencing spontaneous asthma attacks have higher plasma histamine and serotonin levels than nonasthmatic control subjects [13–17].

Recently, lung fibroblasts have been reported to produce eotaxin and are suggested as the major cellular source of eotaxin [9, 10]. We hypothesized that histamine or serotonin might modulate lung fibroblasts to release eotaxin. The results demonstrate that histamine and serotonin stimulate the lung fibroblast cell line (HFL-1) to release eotaxin. These data suggest that these mediators may play a potential role in eosinophil recruitment into the airway.

Materials and Methods

Cell Culture

Human fetal lung fibroblasts (HFL-1, lung, diploid, human, passage 14) were purchased from the American Type Tissue Culture Collection (Rockville, Md., USA). These cells retain features of human lung fibroblast including collagen and fibronectin production [18, 19]. The HFL-1 cells were suspended at 1.0×10^6 cells/ml in Ham's F-12-supplemented penicillin (50 μg/ml; Gibco, Grand Island, N.Y.), streptomycin (50 μg/ml; Gibco), and 10% heat-inactivated fetal bovine serum. Cell suspensions (3 ml) were added to 30-mm diameter tissue culture dishes (Corning, Corning, N.Y., USA) and were cultured at 37 °C in a 5% CO_2 atmosphere. After 2–3 days in culture, the cells had reached confluence and the culture medium was replaced with 2 ml of medium supplemented as above and were incubated one additional day.

Exposure of HFL-1 to Histamine or Serotonin

The culture medium was removed from the cells by washing twice with serum free medium, and cells were incubated in the presence and absence of histamine or serotonin. To determine the dose-dependent release of eotaxin, the cultures were incubated with various concentrations of histamine or serotonin (0, 0.1, 1, 10 and 100 μ*M*, Sigma) at 37 °C in a humidified 5% CO_2 atmosphere for 24 h. Tumor necrosis factor (TNF)-α (10 ng/ml, Sigma) or interleukin (IL)-1β (1 ng/ml, Sigma) were used as positive controls. The time dependent-release of eotaxin was evaluated by incubating HFL-1 for 6–24 h in the presence and absence of histamine (100 μ*M*) or serotonin (100 μ*M*) because this concentration produced the maximal eotaxin stimulation of the doses tested. Cell injury was evaluated by microscopy (cell shape, detachment from tissue culture dish) and trypan blue exclusion. The supernatant fluids were then harvested and stored at –80 °C until assayed.

Measurement of Eotaxin in the Supernatant Fluids

The concentrations of eotaxin were measured in the cell supernatant fluids from HFL-1 using a commercially available ELISA (R&D Systems) according to the manufacturer's instructions. The minimum concentration detected by this method was 15.6 pg/ml.

Evaluation of Eotaxin mRNA Expression

Eotaxin mRNA was analyzed by the reverse transcriptase-polymerase chain reaction (RT-PCR). Total cellular RNA was extracted from adherent cells using a modification of the methods of Chomczynski and Sacchi [20]. The RNA was reverse transcribed using a commercially available kit (Promega). One microgram of the reverse-transcribed DNA was then mixed with Ready to Go PCR Beads (Pharmacia) and the front and back primers added at 0.2 μ*M* final concentration. PCR was performed in a Perkin Elmer model 480 thermal cycler using 94 °C for 2 min and 32 cycles consisting of 94 °C for 45 s, 61 °C for 45 s, 72 °C for 2 min, followed by 72 °C for an additional 7 min. Glyceraldehyde 3-phosphate dehydrogenase (GAPDH) was used as a 'housekeeping gene' with PCR. The DNA was subjected to agarose gel and the intensity of the bands quantitated by densitometry. The results were expressed as the ratio of intensity to the GAPDH. Sequences of the primers were as follows:

Eotaxin (F): 5′-ACATGAAGGTCTCCGCAGCACTTC-3′;
Eotaxin (R): 5′-TTGGCCAGGTTAAAGCAGCAGGTG-3′;
GAPDH (F): 5′-ACCACAGTCCATGCCATCA-3′;
GAPDH (R): 5′-TCCACCACCCTGTTGCTGTA-3′.

Effect of Eotaxin Antibody on Eosinophil Chemotactic Activity by HFL-1 Supernatant Fluids

Eosinophils were isolated with a modified method of Hansel et al. [21] with a magnetic cell separation system (Becton Dickinson). Purity of the eosinophils counted by Randolph's stain was >94%; viability was >98%. The eosinophils were resuspended in Gey's solution at 2.0×10^6 cells/ml and used for the chemotaxis assay.

Eosinophil chemotactic activity (ECA) was assayed in 48-well microchemotaxis chambers (Neuroprobe, Inc., Cabin John, Md., USA) as previously described [22]. The bottom wells of the chamber were filled with 25 μl of the histamine- or serotonin-stimulated HFL-1 supernatant fluids, which were incubated with anti-human eotaxin-neutralizing antibody (R&D systems, 0.1–10 μg/ml) or normal goat Ig-G (R&D systems) for 1 h before chemotactic assay. A 10-μm-thick polyvinylpyrrolidone-free polycarbonate filter with a pore size of 5 μm was placed over the samples. The silicon gasket and the upper pieces of the chamber were applied and 50 μl of the cell suspension was placed into the upper wells. The chambers were incubated in humidified air in 5% CO_2 at 37 °C for 90 min. Nonmigrated cells were wiped away from the filter. The filter was immersed in methanol for 5 min, stained with a modified Wright's stain, and mounted on a glass slide. Cells that had completely migrated through the filter were counted using light microscopy. ECA was expressed as the mean number of migrated cells per high power field from duplicate wells.

Statistics

In experiments where multiple experiments were made, differences between groups were tested for significance using a one way analysis of variance with Duncan's multiple range test applied to data at specific time and dose points. In experiments where single measurements were made, the differences between groups were

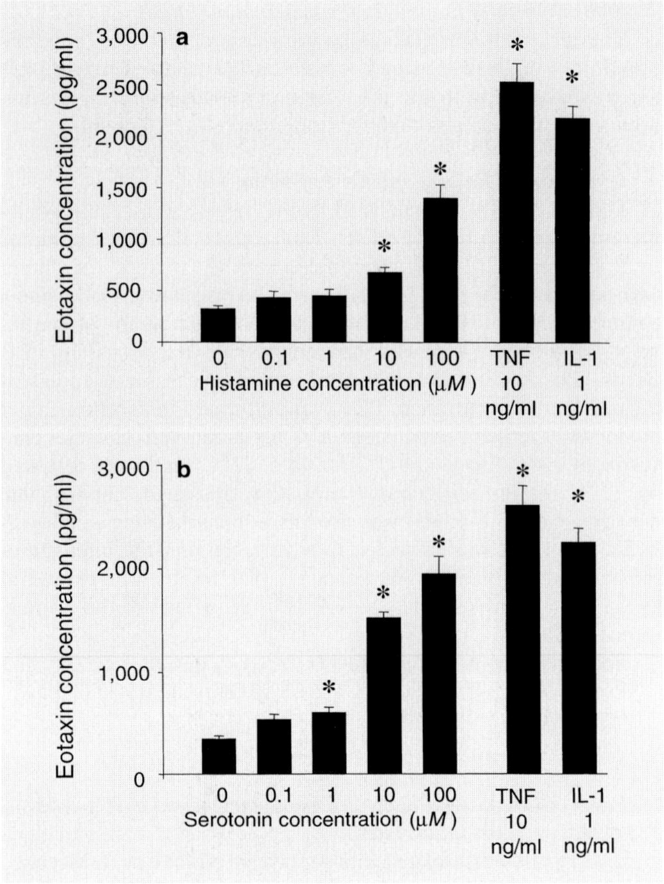

Fig. 1. Dose-dependent release of eotaxin from HFL-1 in response to histamine (**a**) or serotonin (**b**) after 24 h of incubation (n = 5). TNF-α (10 ng/ml) and IL-1β (1 ng/ml) were incubated with HFL-1 to be compared with histamine or serotonin effect. Values are expressed as mean ± SEM. * $p < 0.05$ compared with supernatant fluids without stimulation.

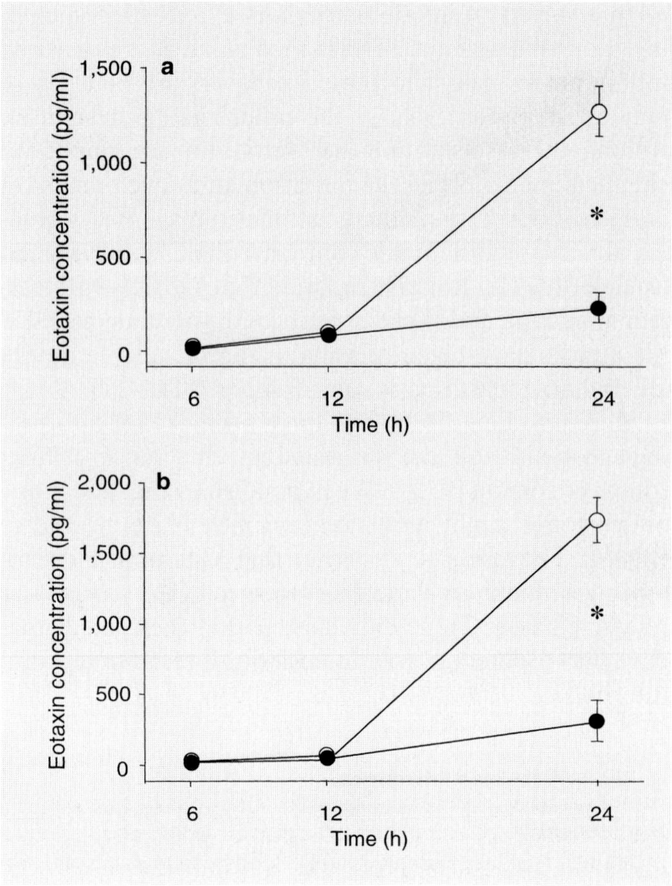

Fig. 2. Time-related release of eotaxin in response to 100 μ*M* of histamine (**a**) or serotonin (**b**) from HFL-1 (n = 4). ○ = Eotaxin release with histamine or serotonin incubation; ● = eotaxin release without stimulation. Values are expressed as mean ± SEM. * $p < 0.05$ compared with supernatant fluids without stimulation.

tested using Student's paired t test. In all cases, a p value of <0.05 was considered significant. Data in figure and tables are expressed as the mean ± SEM.

Results

Release of Eotaxin from HFL-1

HFL-1 released eotaxin spontaneously without stimulation and released eotaxin in a dose-dependent manner in response to histamine or serotonin ($p < 0.05$, fig. 1). The lowest dose of histamine or serotonin to stimulate eotaxin release was 10 or 1.0 μ*M*, respectively. Increasing concentrations of histamine or serotonin progressively increased the release of eotaxin up to 100 μ*M*. Both TNF-α and IL-1β also stimulated the release of eotaxin (fig. 1).

Histamine or serotonin treatment of HFL-1 also resulted in the augmented release of eotaxin in a time-dependent manner ($p < 0.05$, fig. 2). HFL-1 release of eotaxin in response to histamine or serotonin was not significant compared to media alone until 12 h. However, treatment of HFL-1 with histamine (100 μ*M*) or serotonin (100 μ*M*) increased eotaxin release after 24 h.

We also stimulated the lung epithelial cell lines, BEAS 2B cells and A549 cells with histamine or serotonin. The eotaxin concentration by epithelial cell line was below the lower detection limit of the assay (15.6 pg/ml).

Neither histamine nor serotonin caused HFL-1 injury (no deformity of cell shape, no detachment from tissue culture dish, and greater than 95% of cells were viable by trypan blue exclusion) after 24 h of incubation.

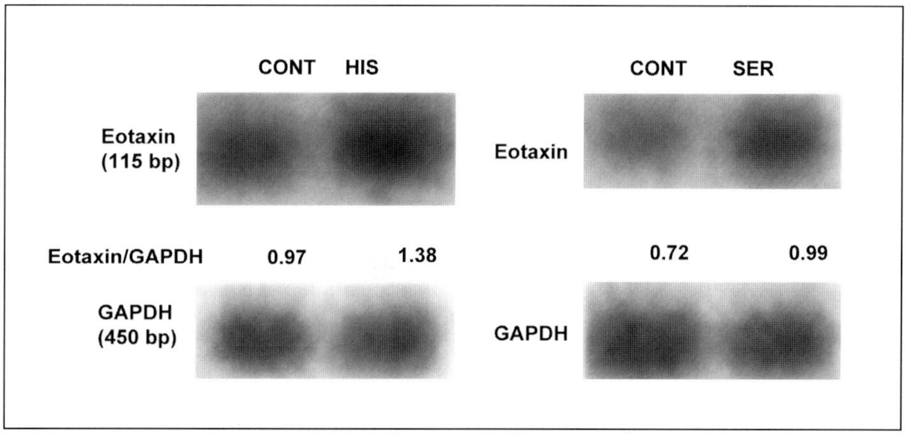

Fig. 3. Augmentation of eotaxin mRNA expression by 100 μ*M* of histamine or serotonin after 12 h of incubation in HFL-1 monolayers. Data are representative of 4 experiments.

Augmentation of Eotaxin mRNA Expression

Histamine or serotonin treatment of HFL-1 for 12 h augmented the expression of eotaxin mRNA (fig. 3).

Inhibition of Eosinophil Chemotactic Activity by Polyclonal Antibody to Eotaxin

HFL-1 released eotaxin spontaneously and histamine or serotonin stimulated the release of eotaxin. Therefore, we evaluated the effect of anti-eotaxin antibody on eosinophil chemotactic activity released into the supernatant fluids by histamine or serotonin-stimulated HFL-1 cells. The anti-eotaxin antibody inhibited eosinophil chemotactic activity induced by the stimulation with histamine or serotonin (100 μ*M*) by about 25 or 30% ($p < 0.05$, fig. 4) but a control antibody did not (fig. 4). Histamine or serotonin itself did not show any ECA (data not shown).

Discussion

The present study demonstrated the spontaneous release of eotaxin by HFL-1 cells. Eotaxin release was significantly augmented in response to histamine or serotonin in a dose- and time-dependent manner. These data suggest that lung fibroblasts may be a major source of eotaxin and play a role in the pathogenesis of asthma by releasing eotaxin in response to these mediators.

There is substantial evidence that injurious agents released from infiltrating eosinophil leukocytes make an important contribution to the airway inflammation characteristic of asthma [1]. However, the precise molecular mechanism of the recruitment of tissue eosinophils remains to be investigated. Eotaxin is directly chemotactic for eosinophils but not mononuclear cells or neutrophils,

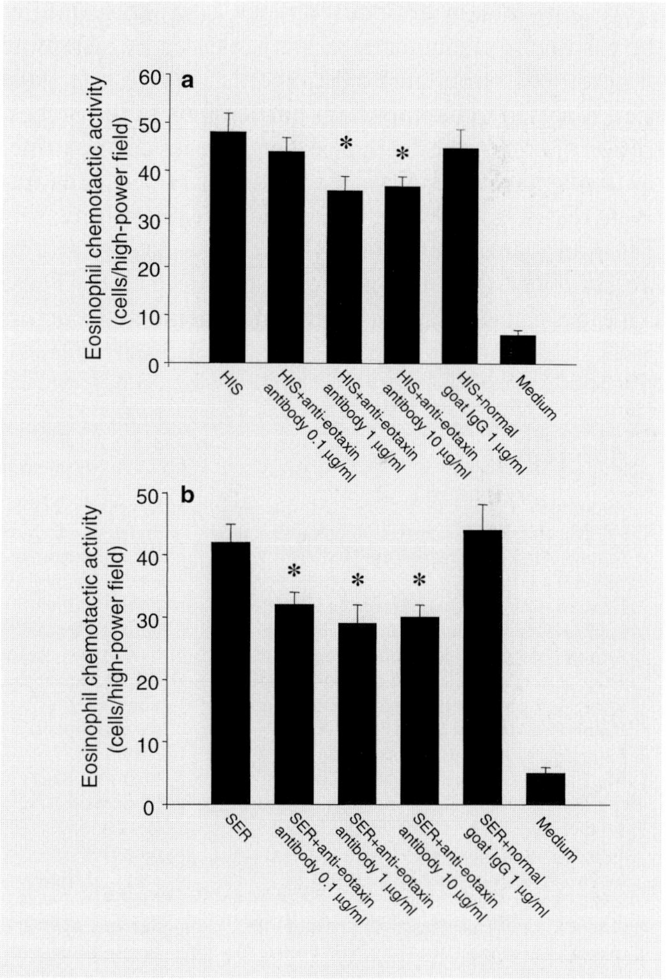

Fig. 4. The effect of anti-eotaxin antibody on eosinophil chemotactic activity released into the supernatant fluids by histamine (**a**)- or serotonin (**b**)-stimulated HFL-1 cells ($n = 4$). Media, Ham's F12 medium alone. Values are expressed as mean ± SEM. * $p < 0.05$ compared with histamine (HIS) or serotonin (SER) treated supernatant fluids.

in addition, airway eotaxin concentrations correlate with the sensitivity of asthmatic airways to contact stimuli [23].

Recently, Teran et al. [9] reported that the amount of immunoreactive eotaxin induced by IL-4 and TNF-α from lung fibroblasts was 3,800–20,000 times greater than that released by cytokine-stimulated A549 epithelial cells. We also stimulated the lung epithelial cell lines, BEAS 2B cells and A549 cells with histamine or serotonin. The eotaxin concentrations in the supernatant fluid of epithelial cell lines were below the lower detection limit of the assay (15.6 pg/ml, data not shown). These observations are consistent with the concept that fibroblasts may be a major source of eotaxin in the lungs and a major source of eosinophil chemotactic activity in allergic airway disorders by releasing eotaxin.

An anti-eotaxin antibody did not completely inhibit the eosinophil chemotactic activity released by histamine or serotonin stimulated HFL-1 cells. Fibroblasts have been reported to be important participants in the orchestration of inflammation by releasing various chemoattractants. We have previously reported that HFL-1 constitutively release granulocyte-macrophage colony-stimulating factor and leukotriene B4 [24], and their concentrations are sufficient to function as chemotactic factors. These cytokines can also serve as eosinophil chemotactic factors and may explain some of the eosinophil chemotactic activity not inhibited by eotaxin antibodies.

As a mediator released by bronchial mast cells or basophils after allergen or nonspecific stimulation [25], histamine is found in greater amounts in BALF from allergic and asthmatic subjects compared to normal subjects. Mast cells are present in densities of 1 to 7 × 10^6 cells/g lung tissue [26], constitute as much as 2% of alveolar tissue [27], and mast cells release histamine upon activation [28]. Histamine concentration in BAL fluid of asthmatic patients after antigen challenge is increased and the concentration is reported to be more than 1 ng/ml [29]. Considering the dilution factors induced by the lavage, the histamine concentration of epithelial lining fluid might be nearly 10 μM which is sufficient to stimulate lung fibroblasts in lung tissue locally after mast cell degranulation. Plasma-free serotonin in symptomatic patients is about 10 ng/ml [30] which is higher than histamine [31] and serotonin concentration in nasal secretion is sometimes higher than 100 nmol/l [32]. Serotonin also may play an important role in inflammatory cell recruitment.

In conclusion, human lung fibroblast cell line, HFL-1, releases eotaxin in response to histamine and serotonin in vitro. These data suggest that histamine and serotonin may play an important role in eosinophil recruitment in allergic airway disorders.

References

1 Bousquet J, Chanez P, Vignola AM, Lacoste JY, Michhel FB: Eosinophil inflammation in asthma. Am J Respir Crit Care Med 1994;150: S33–S38.

2 Okada S, Kita H, George TJ, Gleich GJ, Leiferman KM: Transmigration of eosinophils through basement membrane components in vitro: Synergistic effects of platelet-activating factor and eosinophil-active cytokines. Am J Respir Cell Mol Biol 1997;16:455–463.

3 Gonzalo JA, Lloyd CM, Kremer L, Finger E, Martinez-A C, Siegelman MH, Cybulsky M, Gutierrez-Ramos JC: Eosinophil recruitment to the lung in a murine model of allergic inflammation. The role of T cells, chemokines, and adhesion receptors. J Clin Invest 1996;98: 2332–2345.

4 Jose PJ, Griffiths-Johnson DA, Collins PD, Walsh DT, Moqbel R, Totty NF, Truong O, Hsuan JJ, Williams TJ: Eotaxin: A potent eosinophil chemoattractant cytokine detected in a guinea pig model of allergic airways inflammation. J Exp Med 1994;179:881–887.

5 Daugherty BL, Siciliano SJ, DeMartino JA, Malkowitz L, Sirotina A, Springer MS: Cloning, expression, and characterization of the human eosinophil eotaxin receptor. J Exp Med 1996;183:2349–2354.

6 Ponath PD, Qin S, Post TW, Wang J, Wu L, Gerard NP, Newman W, Gerard C, Mackay CR: Molecular cloning and characterization of a human eotaxin receptor expressed selectively on eosinophils. J Exp Med 1996;183:2437–2448.

7 Mattoli S, Stacey MA, Sun G, Bellini A, Marini M: Eotaxin expression and eosinophilic inflammation in asthma. Biochem Biophys Res Commun 1997;236:299–301.

8 Lilly CM, Nakamura H, Kesselman H, Nagler-Anderson C, Asano K, Garcia-Zepeda EA, Rothenberg ME, Drazen JM, Luster AD: Expression of eotaxin by human lung epithelial cells: Induction by cytokines and inhibition by glucocorticoids. J Clin Invest 1997;99:1767–1773.

9 Teran LM, Mochizuki M, Bartels J, Valencia EL, Nakajima T, Hirai K, Schroder JM: Th1- and Th2-type cytokines regulate the expression and production of eotaxin and RANTES by human lung fibroblasts. Am J Respir Cell Mol Biol 1999;20:777–786.

10 Sato E, Nelson DK, Koyama S, Hoyt JC, Robbins RA: Inflammatory cytokines modulate eotaxin release by human lung fibroblast cell line. Exp Lung Res 2001;27:173–183.

11 White MV, Slater JE, Kaliner MA: Histamine and asthma. Am Rev Respir Dis 1987;135: 1165–1176.

12 Cazzola M, Matera MG, D'Amato G, Rossi F: Effects of serotonin on airways: Recent developments. Allergy 1995;50:1–10.

13 Simon RA, Stevenson DD, Arroyave CM, Tan EM: The relationship of plasma histamine to the activity of bronchial asthma. J Allergy Clin Immunol 1977;60:312–316.

14 Bruce C, Weatherstone R, Seaton A, Taylor WH: Histamine levels in plasma, blood, and urine in severe asthma, and the effect of corticosteroid treatment. Thorax 1976;31:724–729.

15 Barnes PJ, Ind PW, Brown MJ: Plasma histamine and catecholamines in stable asthmatic subjects. Clin Sci 1982;62:661–665.
16 Lechin F, van der Dijs B, Orozco B, Jara H, Rada I, Lechin ME, Lechin AE: The serotonin uptake-enhancing drug tianeptine suppresses asthmatic symptoms in children: A double-blind, crossover, placebo-controlled study. J Clin Pharmacol 1998;38:918–925.
17 Lechin F, van der Dijs B, Orozco B, Lechin M, Lechin AE: Increased levels of free serotonin in plasma of symptomatic asthmatic patients. Ann Allergy Asthma Immunol 1996;77:245–253.
18 Breul SD, Bradley KH, Hance AJ, Schafer MP, Berg RA, Crystal RG: Control of collagen production by human diploid lung fibroblasts. J Biol Chem 1980;255:5250–5260.
19 Katayama K, Seyer JM, Raghow R, Kang AH; Regulation of extracellular matrix production by chemically synthesized subfragments of type I collagen carboxy propeptide. Biochemistry 1991;30:7097–7104.
20 Chomczynski P, Sacchi N. Single-step method of RNA isolation by acid guanidinium thiocyanate-phenol-chloroform extraction. Anal Biochem 1987;162:156–159.
21 Hansel TT, De Vries IJ, Iff T, Rihs S, Wandzilak M, Betz S, Blaser K, Walker C: 1991. An improved immunomagnetic procedure for the isolation of highly purified human blood eosinophils. J Immunol Methods 145:105–110.
22 Harvath L, Falk W, Leonard EJ: Rapid quantification of neutrophil chemotaxis: Use of polyvinylpyrrolidone-free polycarbonate membrane in a multiwell assembly. J Immunol Methods 1980;37:39–45.
23 Ying S, Robinson DS, Meng Q, Rottman J, Kennedy R, Ringler DJ, Mackay CR, Daugherty BL, Springer MS, Durham SR, Williams TJ, Kay AB: Enhanced expression of eotaxin and CCR3 mRNA and protein in atopic asthma. Association with airway hyperresponsiveness and predominant co-localization of eotaxin mRNA to bronchial epithelial and endothelial cells. Eur J Immunol 1997;27:3507–3516.
24 Koyama S, Sato E, Masubuchi T, Takamizawa A, Nomura H, Kubo K, Nagai S, Izumi T: Human lung fibroblasts release chemokinetic activity for monocytes constitutively. Am J Physiol 1998;275:L223–L230.
25 Schleimer RP, Fox CC, Naclerio RM, Plaut M, Creticos PS, Togias AG, Warner JA, Kagey-Sobotka A, Lichtenstein LM: Role of human basophils and mast cells in the pathogenesis of allergic diseases. J Allergy Clin Immunol 1985; 76:369–374.
26 Wasserman SI: The lung mast cell: Its physiology and potential relevance to defense of the lung. Environ Health Perspect 1980;35:153–164.
27 Fox B, Bull TB, Guz A: Mast cells in the human alveolar wall: An electron microscopic study. J Clin Pathol 198; 34:1333–1342.
28 Wasserman SI: Mast cells and airway inflammation in asthma. Am J Respir Crit Care Med 1994;150:S39–S41.
29 Casale TB, Wood D, Richerson HB, Zehr B, Zavala D, Hunninghake GW: Direct evidence of a role for mast cells in the pathogenesis of antigen-induced bronchoconstriction. J Clin Invest 1987;80:1507–1511.
30 Lechin F, van der Dijs B, Orozco B, Lechin M, Lechin AE: Increased levels of free serotonin in plasma of symptomatic asthmatic patients. Ann Allergy Asthma Immunol 1996;77:245–253.
31 Corhay JL, Bury T, Louis R, Radermecker MF: Plasma histamine and bronchial reactivity in allergic asthma. Allergy 1993;48:547–549.
32 Tonnesen P, Hindberg I: Serotonin in nasal secretion. Allergy 1988;43:303–309.

Mini Review

International Archives of Allergy and Immunology

Int Arch Allergy Immunol 2002;128(suppl 1):18–20

Cross-Talk between Integrins and Chemokines That Influences Eosinophil Adhesion and Migration

Hiroshi Tachimoto[a, b] Motohiro Ebisawa[b] Bruce S. Bochner[a]

[a]Department of Medicine, Division of Clinical Immunology, The Johns Hopkins University School of Medicine, Baltimore, Md., USA, and [b]Department of Pediatrics, National Sagamihara Hospital, Kanagawa, Japan

Key Words
Eosinophils · Cell trafficking · Chemokines · Adhesion molecules

Introduction

Eosinophils accumulate selectively at allergic inflammation sites. Numerous studies have been done to clarify the mechanisms of selective eosinophil accumulation during allergic inflammation. Adhesion molecules and chemokines play important roles in selective eosinophil accumulation [1]. For example, eosinophils express $\alpha4\beta1$ integrins, one of the ligands for VCAM-1, but neutrophils do not. Among chemokine receptors, eosinophils express CCR3. Like $\alpha4\beta1$ integrins, CCR3 is not expressed on neutrophils, so its activation effectively and selectively induces eosinophil chemotaxis. In this review, we discuss the regulation of eosinophil integrin function by CCR3-active chemokine.

Expression of Integrins on Eosinophils

Eosinophil recruitment to sites of allergic inflammation is thought to be the result of multiple interactions between endothelial cells and eosinophils involving selective adhesion and migration. Eosinophil migration from within blood vessels into tissue requires several steps such as rolling, tethering, firm adhesion and transendothelial migration. Rolling of eosinophils is thought to be mediated primarily by selectins and their ligands. Rolling of eosinophils on endothelial cells may be followed by the induction of firm adhesion. Firm adhesion and transmigration are mediated by integrins. Integrins have two components: an α and a β subunit. Eosinophils express $\beta1$, $\beta2$ and $\beta7$ integrins [2]. For example, eosinophil $\alpha4\beta1$ integrin binds to VCAM-1 on endothelial cells, which plays an important role in selective eosinophil accumulation on tissue. Interestingly, $\alpha4\beta1$ integrin has not only the ability to mediate firm adhesion but also the ability to participate in rolling on endothelial VCAM-1 under shear conditions in vitro [3], a property shared by $\alpha D\beta2$ integrin [4, 5]. Another ligand of $\alpha4\beta1$ integrin, albeit of lower affinity, is CS-1 peptide, a fragment of fibronectin [6]. The only other $\beta1$ on eosinophils is $\alpha6\beta1$ integrin, a ligand of laminin [7]. Eosinophils also express $\alpha4\beta7$ integrins which bind to the gut-expressed mucosal addressin cell

KARGER
Fax + 41 61 306 12 34
E-Mail karger@karger.ch
www.karger.com

© 2002 S. Karger AG, Basel
1018–2438/02/1285–0018$18.50/0

Accessible online at:
www.karger.com/journals/iaa

Correspondence to: Dr. Hiroshi Tachimoto
National Sagamihara Hospital
18-1 Sakuradai Sagamihara
Kanagawa 228-8522 (Japan)
E-Mail htachimoto@nch.go.jp

adhesion molecule-1 (MAdCAM-1), fibronectin and VCAM-1 [8]. Eosinophils express all four β2 integrins (αLβ2, αMβ2, αXβ2 and αDβ2). Their ligands include intercelluar adhesion molecule-1 (ICAM-1) (αLβ2, αMβ2), ICAM-2 (αLβ2), ICAM-3 (αLβ2, αDβ2), fibrinogen (αMβ2), the complement fragment C3bi (αMβ2, αXβ2), and VCAM-1 (αDβ2) [9].

Expression of Chemokine Receptor on Eosinophil

Eosinophil migration to sites of allergic inflammation is influenced by the presence of chemoattractants. Much effort has been devoted to the identification of selective and potent chemoattractants for eosinophils. The growing list of eosinophil-active chemoattractants includes LTB4, LTD4, LTE4, PAF, C3a and C5a. Although LTD4 and LTE4 induce eosinophil but not neutrophil chemotaxis, many of the other chemoattractants are not selective for eosinophils, and several have, at best, modest activity [10]. As a result, numerous studies have been focused on the chemotactic cytokines termed chemokines and their receptors. Among the numerous known chemokine receptors, eosinophils express CCR1, CCR3, CCR6 and CXCR4 [11, 12]. Perhaps most notable is the expression of CCR3, which binds eotaxin, eotaxin-2, eotaxin-3, MCP-2, MCP-3, MCP-4 and RANTES. Macrophage-derived chemokine (MDC), a CCR4-active chemokine, also induces modest eosinophil chemotaxis [13]. Eosinophils do not express CCR4, so the receptor for MDC on eosinophils remains unknown.

Regulation of Eosinophil Integrin Function by CCR3-Active Chemokines and Other Chemoattractants

Preferential eosinophil accumulation at allergic inflammation sites is the result of interactions involving adhesion molecules, chemokines, and other molecules enabling selective adhesion and detachment events for directed cellular migration. We recently demonstrated that CCR3-active chemokines promote rapid detachment of eosinophils bound to VCAM-1 in vitro [14–16]. Eosinophils adhered well to immobilized human recombinant VCAM-1, primarily via α4β1 integrin. Eotaxin-2, a CCR3-specific chemokine, induced eosinophil de-adhesion from VCAM-1. By contrast, very few eosinophils spontaneously adhered to BSA, and eosinophil adhesion to BSA was enhanced by eotaxin-2 over a similar nanomolar range of concentrations. This enhancement of BSA adhesion was dependent on β2 integrins. The effect of eotaxin-2 on eosinophil adhesion to VCAM-1 and BSA occurred within 3 min and was sustained for at least 60 min. Similar effects were seen with other chemoattractants, such as RANTES and PAF. The reduction of eosinophil adhesion to VCAM-1 and the enhancement of eosinophil adhesion to BSA by eotaxin-2 was prevented by a CCR3-blocking mAb.

Integrins on eosinophils exist in high- and low-affinity states [6, 17]. To explore the mechanism by which chemokines affect adhesion, the effect of chemokines or integrin expression was determined [14]. Levels of α4 and β1 integrin expression on eosinophils were unchanged or slightly decreased by eotaxin-2 treatment. More impressive was the finding that levels of the activated β1 integrin epitope were remarkably decreased. It appears likely, therefore, that the reduction of eosinophil adhesion to VCAM-1 in response to eotaxin-2 was primarily due to changes in β1 integrin function rather than expression.

Eosinophil α4β1 integrins can mediate rolling on VCAM-1 under physiological flow conditions [3, 5]. Although we observed a reduction of eosinophil accumulation on immobilized VCAM-1 in response to eotaxin-2 under physiological flow conditions, this reduction of adhesion was not observed when both VCAM-1 and ICAM-1 were co-immobilized [18]. Based on antibody-blocking studies, this appears to be due to a chemokine-induced shift in integrin usage away from β1 integrin-dominated interactions with VCAM-1 toward β2 integrin-dominated interactions with ICAM-1. In some ways, our results seem to differ from some previous reports. Our data showed that CCR3-active chemokine activated eosinophil β2 integrin function, a result consistent with the work of others [15, 16, 19]. However, it was reported that chemokines and C5a activated α4β1 integrin only transiently, followed by subsequent inhibition [15, 20]. Others have reported that maximally activated adhesion, induced through β1 integrins with a unique integrin-activating mAb, actually inhibited eosinophil transmigration by preventing cell movement [21]. Furthermore, eosinophil migration across human pulmonary microvascular endothelial cells inversely correlated with eosinophil adhesion and VCAM-1 expression [22]. These data suggest that activation of β1 integrins can inhibit migration and that chemokines downregulate β1 integrin function during eosinophil migration.

Conclusion

Our results confirm the important role of integrins and chemokines in selective eosinophil migration processes. CCR3-active chemokines may be necessary to facilitate de-adhesion from luminal VCAM-1 as well as the process of diapedesis by shifting integrin usage in eosinophils away from β1 integrin-dominated interactions with VCAM-1 towards β2 integrin-dominated interactions with ICAM-1. The critical importance of integrins and chemokines in eosinophilic inflammation lends support to the idea of targeting these molecules with novel therapeutic agents.

References

1 Wardlaw AJ: Molecular basis for selective eosinophil trafficking in asthma: A multistep paradigm (review). J Allergy Clin Immunol 1999; 104:917–926.
2 Tachimoto H, Bochner BS: The surface phenotype of human eosinophils (review); in Marone G (ed): Human Eosinophils: Biologic and Clinical Aspects. Chem Immunol. Basel, Karger, 2000, vol 76, pp 45–62.
3 Sriramarao P, von Andrian UH, Butcher EC, Bourdon MA, Broide DH: L-selectin and very late antigen-4 integrin promote eosinophil rolling at physiological shear rates in vivo. J Immunol 1994;153:4238–4246.
4 Grayson MH, Van der Vieren M, Sterbinsky SA, et al: αdβ2 integrin is expressed on human eosinophils and functions as an alternative ligand for vascular cell adhesion molecule 1 (VCAM-1). J Exp Med 1998;188:2187–2191.
5 Kikuchi M, Tachimoto M, Hudson SA, Bochner BS: Phorbol myristate acetate (PMA) alters human eosinophil expression of α4β1 and αdβ2 integrins and adhesion to VCAM-1 under static and flow conditions (abstract). J Allergy Clin Immunol. 2000;105:S258.
6 Matsumoto K, Sterbinsky SA, Bickel CA, Zhou DW, Kovach NL, Bochner BS: Regulation of α4 integrin-mediated adhesion of human eosinophils to fibronectin and vascular cell adhesion molecule-1 (VCAM-1). J Allergy Clin Immunol 1997;99:648–656.
7 Georas SN, McIntyre BW, Ebisawa M, et al: Expression of a functional laminin receptor (α6 β1, very late activation antigen-6) on human eosinophils. Blood 1993;82:2872–2879.
8 Walsh GM, Symon FA, Lazarovits AI, Wardlaw AJ: Integrin α4β7 mediates human eosinophil interaction with MAdCAM-1, VCAM-1 and fibronectin. Immunology 1996;89:112–119.
9 Davenpeck K, Bochner BS: Leukocyte-blood vessel interactions; in Zweiman B, Schwartz LB (eds): Inflammatory Mechanisms in Allergic Disease. New York, Marcel Dekker, 2002, pp 125–141.
10 Broide D, Sriramarao P: Eosinophil trafficking to sites of allergic inflammation. Immunol Rev 2001;179:163–172.
11 Nagase H, Miyamasu M, Yamaguchi M, et al: Expression of CXCR4 in eosinophils: Functional analyses and cytokine-mediated regulation. J Immunol 2000;164:5935–5943.
12 Sullivan SK, McGrath DA, Liao F, Boehme SA, Farber JM, Bacon KB: MIP-3α induces human eosinophil migration and activation of the mitogen-activated protein kinases (p42/p44 MAPK). J Leukoc Biol 1999;66:674–682.
13 Bochner BS, Bickel CA, Taylor ML, et al: Macrophage-derived chemokine induces human eosinophil chemotaxis in a CC chemokine receptor 3- and CC chemokine receptor 4-independent manner. J Allergy Clin Immunol 1999; 103:527–532.
14 Tachimoto H, Burdick MM, Hudson SA, Kikuchi M, Konstantopoulos K, Bochner BS: CCR3-active chemokines promote rapid detachment of eosinophils from VCAM-1 in vitro. J Immunol 2000;165:2748–2754.
15 Weber C, Katayama J, Springer TA: Differential regulation of β1 and β2 integrin avidity by chemoattractants in eosinophils. Proc Natl Acad Sci USA 1996;93:10939–10944.
16 Sung KP, Yang L, Kim J, et al: Eotaxin induces a sustained reduction in the functional adhesive state of very late antigen 4 for the connecting segment 1 region of fibronectin. J Allergy Clin Immunol 2000;106:933–940.
17 Werfel SJ, Yednock TA, Matsumoto K, Sterbinsky SA, Schleimer RP, Bochner BS: Functional regulation of β1 integrins on human eosinophils by divalent cations and cytokines. Am J Respir Cell Mol Biol 1996;14:44–52.
18 Tachimoto H, Hudson SA, Bochner BS: Eotaxin-2 rapidly shifts eosinophil integrin usage from β1 integrin/VCAM-1-dominated interactions to β2 integrin/ICAM-1-dominated interactions (abstract). J Allergy Clin Immunol 2001;107:S734.
19 Nagata M, Yamamoto H, Tabe K, Sakamoto Y: Eosinophil transmigration across VCAM-1-expressing endothelial cells is upregulated by antigen-stimulated mononuclear cells. Int Arch Allergy Immunol 2001;125(suppl 1):7–11.
20 Kitayama J, Mackay CR, Ponath PD, Springer TA: The C-C chemokine receptor CCR3 participates in stimulation of eosinophil arrest on inflammatory endothelium in shear flow. J Clin Invest 1998;101:2017–2024.
21 Kuijpers TW, Mul EP, Blom M, et al: Freezing adhesion molecules in a state of high-avidity binding blocks eosinophil migration. J Exp Med 1993;178:279–284.
22 Yamamoto H, Sedgwick JB, Busse WW: Differential regulation of eosinophil adhesion and transmigration by pulmonary microvascular endothelial cells. J Immunol 1998;161:971–977.

Mini Review

International Archives of Allergy and Immunology

Int Arch Allergy Immunol 2002;128(suppl 1):21–23

Potential Initiation of Eosinophilic Skin Inflammation by Antigen-Specific T Helper Type 2 Cells

Osamu Kaminuma[a, b] Akio Mori[a]

[a]Clinical Research Center for Allergy and Rheumatology, National Sagamihara Hospital, Kanagawa, and
[b]Department of Immunology, The Tokyo Metropolitan Institute of Medical Science, Tokyo, Japan

Key Words
Th2 cells · Eosinophils · Atopic dermatitis

This review focuses on a specific aspect of the pathogenesis of atopic dermatitis: the role of Th2 cells in eosinophilic inflammation. Growing evidence suggests that eosinophils actively participate in the development of atopic dermatitis [1]. Extensive deposits of extracellular eosinophil major basic protein have been observed in allergic lesional skin [2]. Disease activity of atopic dermatitis correlates with eosinophil numbers and/or eosinophil cationic protein concentrations [3]. Eosinophil granule proteins demonstrate potent cytotoxic activity [4], suggesting that eosinophils are contributing to dermal tissue damage in atopic dermatitis.

IgE is also an important component of atopic dermatitis, and one that distinguishes it from the other nonallergic diseases [5]. Serum IgE levels are elevated in 80–85% of patients with atopic dermatitis. Approximately 85% of patients show positive immediate skin test or RAST results for specific IgE in response to a variety of food allergens [6]. When IgE-bearing mast cells are directed to the relevant antigen, they release eosinophil-acting mediators including IL-3, IL-4, IL-5, IL-13, TNF-α, and GM-CSF [7]. The involvement of IgE in peripheral tissue eosinophilia has also been demonstrated using animal models of allergic inflammation [8].

In the development of atopic dermatitis, Th2 cells play a crucial role in both eosinophil activation and IgE synthesis. The number of CD4+ T cells is increased in the lesional skin and peripheral blood of patients with atopic dermatitis [9]. CD4+ T cells infiltrated in dermal tissues appear to have a Th2 phenotype [10]. IL-5, a Th2 cytokine, promotes terminal differentiation of the committed eosinophil precursors, eosinophil activation and chemotaxis, and prolongs the survival of eosinophils [11]. Another Th2 cytokine, IL-4, is an essential factor for IgE production as it stimulates transcription at the Cε locus in B cells. This locus contains the exons responsible for encoding the constant-region domains of the IgE ε-heavy chain [12]. Together, Th2 cells orchestrate the development of eosinophilic inflammation in atopic dermatitis by activating eosinophils directly as well as through an IgE/mast cell-dependent cascade.

However, the relative contribution of IgE/mast cell-dependent and -independent mechanisms to the accumulation of eosinophils in atopic dermatitis is still controversial. This is partly due to the fact that there are few good animal models of atopic dermatitis. Dermal eosinophilic inflammation is not obvious in 'classic' models of skin

KARGER
Fax +41 61 306 12 34
E-Mail karger@karger.ch
www.karger.com

© 2002 S. Karger AG, Basel
1018–2438/02/1285–0021$18.50/0

Accessible online at:
www.karger.com/journals/iaa

Correspondence to: Dr. Osamu Kaminuma
Department of Immunology
The Tokyo Metropolitan Institute of Medical Science
3-18-22 Honkomagome, Bunkyo-ku, Tokyo 113-8613 (Japan)
Tel./Fax +81 3 5685 6608, E-Mail kaminuma@rinshoken.or.jp

diseases, such as passive cutaneous anaphylaxis, delayed-type hypersensitivity and Arthus reaction. In 1997, the development of atopic dermatitis-like skin inflammation was reported in NC/Nga mice [13]. The inflammation had occurred spontaneously on face, neck, ears and dorsal skin under conventional circumstances and, most importantly, eosinophils had massively infiltrated inflamed skin tissues [13]. More detailed analyses using NC/Nga mice may provide useful clues for understanding the pathogenesis of atopic dermatitis. However, this model did not allow Matsuda et al. [13] to distinguish between IgE/mast cell-dependent and independent pathways, since the skin inflammation in NC/Nga mice was accompanied by IgE hyperproduction.

Recently, the direct action of T cells on eosinophilic inflammation has been successfully distinguished from the IgE/mast cell system by using an animal model of asthma. Eosinophilic inflammation was triggered in the lungs of normal mice, despite the absence of antigen-specific IgE, by transferring in vitro-differentiated antigen-specific Th2 cells [14, 15]. Eosinophilic infiltration into the airways of these mice, occurred upon inhalation challenge with the relevant antigen, is dependent on IL-5, but not IL-4 produced by infused T cells. The intensity of eosinophilic accumulation correlates with that of the bronchial hyperresponsiveness to acetylcholine [15]. In addition, the accumulation of antigen-specific Th2 cells in the lungs was required for the subsequent infiltration of eosinophils [16].

T cells as well as eosinophils utilize a variety of adhesion molecules and chemokine-chemokine receptor pairs for the infiltration towards peripheral tissues. The interaction with VCAM-1- and ICAM-1-expressing vascular endothelial cells is essential for the migration of both T cells and eosinophils [16, 17]. The expression of VCAM-1 and ICAM-1 is upregulated in allergic subjects and mediated, at least in part, by Th2 cytokines [17]. Enhanced expression of C-C chemokines, eotaxin, and regulated on activation, normal T cell expressed and secreted (RANTES) has been demonstrated in skin biopsies from patients with atopic dermatitis. Accordingly, both Th2 cells and eosinophils highly express their counter receptor, the C-C chemokine receptor 3 (CCR3) [18].

Most recently, it was found that for inducing eosinophilic inflammation, Th2 cells do not only target the lungs, but also the skin [Kaminuma et al., unpublished observations]. This finding is interesting, because the homing of Th2 cells towards the skin, which is a prerequisite for the subsequent eosinophilic infiltration, has been reported to be dependent on their special characteristics. For example, cutaneous lymphocyte-associated antigen (CLA) is thought to be involved in the selective direction of memory T cells to cutaneous inflammatory sites. In peripheral blood of atopic dermatitis, Th2 cells in CLA+ cell populations are significantly increased, whereas CLA+ Th1 cells are decreased [19]. Chemoattractant receptor-homologous molecules expressed on Th2 cells (CRTH2) were recently identified as a novel G protein-coupled receptor. They are selectively expressed in Th2 (but not in Th1) cells, and they are highly expressed on circulating T cells of atopic dermatitis [20]. Further, thymus and activation-regulated chemokine (TARC) and macrophage-derived chemokine (MDC) was specifically expressed in the inflamed skin of NC/Nga mice, and the expression was associated with disease activity [21]. T cells accumulating in the skin highly expressed their counter receptor, CCR4, accordingly [21]. The cell transfer procedure described above may be useful to evaluate the exact roles of those skin-specific molecules in the initiation of dermal eosinophilic inflammation.

In summary, Th2 cells can directly regulate eosinophilic inflammation in atopic dermatitis, independent of the IgE/mast cell system. Further work to elucidate the mechanism of allergic inflammation, including the IgE/mast cell system, will help us to focus on the most convincing targets for therapeutic intervention of allergic diseases.

References

1 Leiferman KM: Eosinophils in atopic dermatitis. J Allergy Clin Immunol 1994;94:1310–1317.

2 Ott NL, Gleich GJ, Peterson EA, Fujisawa T, Sur S, Leiferman KM: Assessment of eosinophil and neutrophil participation in atopic dermatitis: Comparison with the IgE-mediated late phase reaction. J Allergy Clin Immunol 1994;94:120–128.

3 Kagi MK, Joller-Jemelka H, Wüthrich B: Correlation of eosinophils, eosinophils cationic protein and soluble interleukin-2 receptor with the clinical activity of atopic dermatitis. Dermatology 1992;185:88–92.

4 Walsh GM: Eosinophil granule proteins and their role in disease. Curr Opin Hematol 2001;8:28–33.

5 Broide DH: Molecular and cellular mechanisms of allergic disease (review). J Allergy Clin Immunol 2001;108 (suppl 2):S65–S71.

6 Sampson HA, Albergo R: Comparison of results of skin tests, RAST, and double-blind, placebo controlled food challenges in children with atopic dermatitis. J Allergy Clin Immunol 1984;74:26–33.

7 Gordon JR, Burd PR, Galli SJ: Mast cells as source of multifunctional cytokines. Immunol Today 1990;11:458–464.

8 Coyle AJ, Wagner K, Bertrand C, Tsuyuki S, Bews J, Heusser C: Central role of immunoglobulin (Ig) E in the induction of lung eosinophil infiltration and T helper 2 cell cytokine production: Inhibition by a non-anaphylactogenic anti-IgE antibody. J Exp Med 1996;183:1303–1320.

9 Lever DYM, Turbitt M, Sanderson A, MacKie R: Immunophenotyping of the cutaneous infiltrate and of the mononuclear cells in the peripheral blood in patients with atopic dermatitis. J Invest Dermatol 1987;89:4–7.

10 Romagnani S: Human TH1 and TH2 subsets: Doubt no more. Immunol Today 1991;12:256–257.

11 Hamelmann E, Gelfand EW: IL-5-induced airway eosinophilia – the key to asthma? (Review). Immunol Rev 2001;179:182–191.

12 Oettgen HC, Geha RS: IgE in asthma and atopy: Cellular and molecular connections. J Clin Invest 1999;104:829–835.

13 Matsuda H, Watanabe N, Geba GP, Sperl J, Tsudzuki M, Hiroi J, Matsumoto M, Ushio H, Saito S, Askenase PW, Ra C: Development of atopic dermatitis-like skin lesion with IgE hyperproduction in NC/Nga mice. Int Immunol 1997;9:461–466.

14 Kaminuma O, Mori A, Ogawa K, Nakata A, Kikkawa H, Naito K, Suko M, Okudaira H: Successful transfer of late phase eosinophil infiltration in the lung by infusion of helper T cell clones. Am J Respir Cell Mol Biol 1997;16:448–454.

15 Nakata A, Kaminuma O, Ogawa K, Fujimura H, Fushimi K, Kikkawa H, Naito K, Ikezawa K, Egan RW, Mori A: Correlation between eosinophilia induced by CD4+ T cells and bronchial hyperresponsiveness. Int Immunol 2001;13:329–339.

16 Kaminuma O, Fujimura H, Fushimi K, Nakata A, Sakai A, Chishima S, Ogawa K, Kikuchi M, Kikkawa H, Akiyama K, Mori A: Dynamics of antigen-specific helper T cells at the initiation of airway eosinophilic inflammation. Eur J Immunol 2001;31:2669–2679.

17 Meager A: Cytokine regulation of cellular adhesion molecule expression in inflammation (Review). Cytokine Growth Factor Rev 1999;10:27–39.

18 Parnia S, Frew AJ: Chemokines and atopic dermatitis. J Allergy Clin Immunol 2000;105:892–894.

19 Teraki Y, Hotta T, Shiohara T: Increased circulating skin-homing cutaneous lymphocyte-associated antigen (CLA)+ type 2 cytokine-producing cells, and decreased CLA+ type 1 cytokine-producing cells in atopic dermatitis. Br J Dermatol 2000;143:373–378.

20 Suenobu N, Kweon M, Kiyono H: Role of chemokine in mucosal disease and dermatitis. Mol Med (Japanese) 2001;38:144–151.

21 Vestergaard C, Yoneyama H, Murai M, Nakamura K, Tamaki K, Terashima Y, Imai T, Yoshie O, Irimura T, Mizutani H, Matsushima K: Overproduction of Th2-specific chemokines in NC/Nga mice exhibiting atopic dermatitis-like lesions. J Clin Invest 1999;104:1097–1105.

International Archives of Allergy and Immunology

Int Arch Allergy Immunol 2002;128(suppl 1):24–27

Airway Epithelial Cells Promote Transmigration of Eosinophils in a New Three-Dimensional Chemotaxis Model

Yoshiko Kato[a], Takao Fujisawa[b], Michiko Shibano[c], Takuya Saito[d], Wataru Gatto[b], Hitoshi Kamiya[b], Koichi Hirai[e], Michihiro Sumida[f], Osamu Yoshie[c]

[a] Department of Psychiatry, University of Mie School of Medicine, Tsu, [b] Department of Pediatrics and Allergy, National Mie Hospital, Tsu, [c] Department of Microbiology, Kinki University School of Medicine, Osaka, [d] Department of Biotechnological Science, Kinki University School of Biology-Oriented Science and Technology, Wakayama, [e] Department of Bioregulatory Function, University of Tokyo, School of Medicine, Tokyo, [f] Department of Second Medical Biochemistry, Ehime University School of Medicine, Shigenobu, Ehime, Japan

Prominent infiltration of eosinophils (EOSs) in the airway mucosa is the pathognomonic sign of asthma. The role of airway epithelial cells in EOS infiltration, however, has not been fully elucidated. The aim of this study is to develop a new in vitro transmigration system composed of airway epithelial cells and extracellular matrix, and to investigate the role of airway epithelial cells in EOS infiltration. A layer of type I collagen gel was formed in Netwell™, and BEAS-2B bronchial epithelial cells were cultured on the gel. Then, the wells covered with an epithelial monolayer were filled with medium, inverted, and new upper chambers were constructed on the gel side by applying a ring cap. After further incubation with or without exogenous cytokines for 48 h, EOSs or neutrophils were loaded in the upper chambers (gel side) and the cells that had transmigrated to the lower chambers (the epithelial cell side) were counted. Immunohistochemical analyses were also performed. While a simple collagen gel hardly promoted EOS migration even in the presence of eotaxin or RANTES, significant numbers of EOSs migrated to lower chambers in the presence of the epithelial cells. Replacement of medium in the lower chamber (epithelial cell side) with fresh medium, addition of exogenous eotaxin or RANTES in the upper chamber (gel side), or pretreatment of EOSs with anti-CCR3 all inhibited transmigration. We found that the epithelial cells produced and deposited extracellular matrix proteins such as type IV collagen onto the type I collagen gel. Separately, we found that type IV collagen itself was capable of enhancing eotaxin-induced EOS migration in a standard chemotaxis assay. Neutrophils also efficiently migrated in the present transmigration system. Pretreatment of epithelial cells with TNF-α and IL-4 enhanced EOS transmigration, while transmigration of neutrophils was enhanced by TNF-α but suppressed by IL-4. In conclusion, by utilizing a new in vitro transmigration system mimicking the airway mucosa, we have demonstrated that airway epithelial cells play an essential role in the transmigration of EOSs and that multiple factors such as chemokines, extracellular matrix proteins and exogenous inflammatory cytokines are involved in efficient transmigration (Clin Exp Allergy, in press).

Eosinophil Transendothelial Migration Induced by Bronchoalveolar Lavage Fluid from Acute Eosinophilic Pneumonia

Hisakazu Shoda, Makoto Nagata, Tetsu Shirai, Keiko Saitou, Hideaki Yamamoto, Yoshio Sakamoto

Pulmonary Division, Second Department of Internal Medicine, Saitama Medical School, Saitama, Japan

Acute eosinophilic pneumonia (AEP) is an idiopathic cause of respiratory distress, characterized by a massive pulmonary infiltration of eosinophils (EOSs). The mechanisms regulating the selective accumulation of EOSs in AEP have not been fully delineated; however, factor(s) produced in the disease sites are likely implicated in the pathophysiology of the disease. In the present study, we examined whether bronchoalveolar lavage fluid (BALF) obtained from patients with AEP regulates transendothelial migration (TM) of blood EOSs in vitro. EOSs were isolated from blood of healthy subjects and placed on the human pulmonary microvascular endothelial cell (HPMEC) monolayers cultured on transwell filter (3 μm pore size). Saline (control) or BALF from patients with AEP or hypersensitivity pneumonitis (HP) was applied to the lower compartment and then TM of EOSs was examined. The BALF from AEP significantly promoted EOS TM across resting HPMEC (%TM: 3.6 ± 1.2 by control, 4.8 ± 2.6 by BALF of HP vs. 17.8 ± 3.1 by BALF of AEP, $p < 0.001$, n = 8). To test whether the expression of VCAM-1 modify the TM induced by BALF of AEP, HPMEC were cultured with IL-4 plus TNF-α (both 100 p*M*, 24 h) and then TM was examined: the TM was not modified. TM induced by BALF of AEP was blocked by an anti-β2 integrin, but not by anti-α4 integrin mAb. Finally, anti-CCR3 antibody had little effect on the TM induced by BALF of AEP. These results suggest that factor(s) other than CC chemokines are produced at the disease site and are responsible for EOS TM in AEP. The factor(s) does not require the interaction of α4 integrin/VCAM-1 in the development of TM.

Leukotriene D_4 Augments Eosinophil Adhesion via Cys LT1-Receptor

Makoto Nagata, Keiko Saitou, Hideaki Yamamoto, Yoshio Sakamoto

Pulmonary Division, Second Department of Internal Medicine, Saitama Medical School, Saitama, Japan

Eosinophils (EOSs) are the major source of cysteinyl leukotriene (cys LT) in allergic inflammation. There is evidence that cys LT_1 receptor antagonists exert modest anti-inflammatory effects in the asthmatic airway in vivo. Although the exact mechanism of this effect remains unknown, cys LT may regulate the cellular responses involved in allergic inflammation. For example, it has been shown that LTD_4 augments the chemotactic response or the survival of

KARGER

Fax + 41 61 306 12 34
E-Mail karger@karger.ch
www.karger.com

© 2002 S. Karger AG, Basel
1018–2438/02/1285–0024$18.50/0

Accessible online at:
www.karger.com/journals/iaa

EOSs. The present study was undertaken to examine whether LTD_4 modified the adhesive properties of EOSs. EOSs were isolated from blood of healthy subjects. Adhesion of EOSs to plastic, rh-ICAM-1, or rh-VCAM-1 was examined in the presence or absence of LTD_4. LTD_4 significantly augmented EOS adhesion to plastic (% adhesion: 5.4 ± 0.8 by medium control vs. 8.0 ± 0.7 by 100 n*M* LTD_4, $p < 0.01$, n = 5). Moreover, LTD_4 augmented EOS adhesion to rh-ICAM-1. On the other hand, EOS adhesion to rh-VCAM-1 was not modified by LTD_4. Flow cytometry analysis revealed that LTD_4 significantly enhanced the expression of CD11b and CD18 on EOS surface. Finally, the enhanced EOS adhesion by LTD_4 was blocked by pranlukast, a cys LT_1 receptor antagonist. These results suggest that LTD_4 directly upregulates the adhesive properties of EOSs via cys LT_1 receptor and β_2 integrin. LTD_4 released from EOSs, or other inflammatory cells, may contribute to the development of EOS accumulation in the asthmatic airway.

CC Chemokines as Augmentative Agents for Eosinophil Adhesion

Norihiro Saito[a], Yoshiyuki Yamada[b], Satoshi Sannohe[b], Cui Chang-Hao[b], Akira Kanda[b], Kazutoshi Yamaguchi[b], Kazuyuki Hamada[b], Junichi Chihara[a,b]

[a]Division of Central Laboratory, Akita University Hospital and [b]Department of Clinical and Laboratory Medicine, Akita University School of Medicine, Akita, Japan

Adhesion molecules and CC chemokines are believed to play an important role in the accumulation of EOSs in allergic inflammation. We observed that both RANTES and eotaxin augmented EOS adhesion to plates coated with r-sICAM-1 without any upregulated expression of β2 integrins. Pertussis toxin, wortmannin and genistein inhibited chemokine-induced adherence. Moreover, we observed that both CCR3 antagonist and CCR1,3 dual antagonist inhibited the functional augmentation of EOS adhesion and intracellular tyrosine phosphorylation of EOSs induced by RANTES or eotaxin. Thus, RANTES and eotaxin are closely related to EOS accumulation not only as chemotactic agents but also as augmentative agents for EOS adhesion through involvement in functional EOS adherence as well as in surface expression of adhesion molecules on EOSs. This could be an important mechanism for the regulation of EOS accumulation and function in the inflammatory sites.

Effect of Dexamethasone on Eosinophilopoiesis from Human Umbilical Cord Blood Mononuclear Cells Stimulated by IL-5

Masato Muraki[a], Yuji Tohda[a], Masahiro Fukuoka[a], Shigenori Nakajima[b], Hirohito Kita[c], Gerald J. Gleich[c]

[a]Fourth Department of Internal Medicine, Kinki University School of Medicine, Osakasayama, Osaka, and [b]Nara Hospital, Kinki University School of Medicine, Ikoma, Nara, Japan; [c]Department of Medicine and Immunology, Mayo Clinic and Foundation, Rochester, Minn., USA

EOSs cause allergic inflammation and play an important role in allergic diseases. Glucocorticosteroids have been used as anti-inflammatory drugs for a long time. In this study, the effect of dexamethasone on eosinophilopoiesis produced from human umbilical cord blood mononuclear cells (UCMC) stimulated by interleukin-5 (IL-5) was investigated. UCMC were cultured with IL-5 (5 ng/ml) on culture plates for 4 weeks. The numbers, morphology of cultured cells and both EOS-derived neurotoxin (EDN) and EOS peroxidase (EPO) in cell lysate were evaluated once a week for 4 weeks. The number of eosinophilic myelocytes and EDN and EPO content in cultured cells increased weekly in the presence of IL-5 (control). On day 8, the numbers of eosinophilic myelocytes decreased slightly under dexamethasone; however, there were no differences in EOS numbers between control and dexamethasone-treated groups from day 15. Although EOSs showed subtle differences in numbers, EDN and EPO content in cultured cells stimulated by IL-5 decreased significantly ($p < 0.05$) under dexamethasone. These results suggested that dexamethasone might suppress EOS maturation. Dexamethasone is useful for the therapy on allergic diseases having EOSs as a central force.

Chemokine Receptor Expression Profile of Eosinophils at Inflamed Tissue Sites: Decreased CCR3 and Increased CXCR4 Expression by Lung Eosinophils

Hiroyuki Nagase[a], Koichiro Kudo[e], Shinyu Izumi[e], Ken Ohta[f], Nobuyuki Kobayashi[e], Masao Yamaguchi[b], Kouji Matsushima[c], Yutaka Morita[a], Kazuhiko Yamamoto[b], Koichi Hirai[d]

Departments of [a]Respiratory Medicine, [b]Allergy and Rheumatology, [c]Molecular Preventive Medicine and CREST, and [d]Bioregulatory Function, University of Tokyo Graduate School of Medicine, Tokyo, [e]Department of Pulmonology, International Medical Center of Japan, Tokyo, and [f]Department of Internal Medicine, Teikyo University School of Medicine, Tokyo, Japan

Most studies dealing with eosinophil (EOS) chemokine receptors (CRs) have employed EOSs isolated from peripheral blood (PB). Although, during the movement of EOSs from the PB to inflamed tissue sites, microenvironmental signals may alter their expression of CRs, little is known about their expression profile at inflamed tissue sites. To determine whether EOSs that have migrated into inflamed tissues exhibit a profile of CR expression different from that in peripheral locations, we simultaneously studied the expression and function of CRs in both BALF and PB specimens of 7 patients with eosinophilic lung disease. De novo expression of CCR2, CCR4 and CCR5 was not detected at either the protein or the mRNA level. However, surface CCR3 expression was decreased and CXCR4 was conversely increased in BALF EOSs and these changes were reflected in the altered migratory response. On the other hand, the levels of CXCR1, CXCR2, CXCR3 and CCR1 were virtually unchanged in BALF EOSs and had no functional significance. In conclusion, EOSs at inflamed tissue sites exhibited an expression profile qualitatively similar to that in peripheral locations, except for a decreased CCR3 and an increased CXCR4 expression. Our results suggest that CCR3 is primarily and CXCR4 is cooperatively involved in EOS accumulation at inflamed tissue sites (J Allergy Clin Immunol 2001;108:563–569).

Respiratory Syncytial Virus Binds to Human Eosinophils and Enhances Expression of CD11b Molecules and the Generation of Superoxide Anion Primed with Platelet-Activating Factor

Masahiko Kato[a], Hirokazu Kimura[b], Atsushi Tachibana[a], Toru Fujiu[a], Masato Suzuki[a], Hiroyuki Mochizuki[a], Kenichi Tokuyama[a], Akihiro Morikawa[a]

[a]Department of Pediatrics, Gunma University, School of Medicine, and [b]Gunma Prefectural Institute of Public Health and Environmental Sciences, Maebashi, Japan

Respiratory syncytial virus (RSV) infection in infancy and early childhood causes acute bronchiolitis and exacerbates bronchial asthma. Eosinophil (EOS) infiltration may contribute to airway obstruction in RSV infection. Our goal was to investigate whether RSV affects EOS function. Binding of RSV to EOSs was assessed by direct immunofluorescence. EOS activation was evaluated by chemiluminescent detection of superoxide anion (O_2^-) generation. Expression of CD11b on EOSs was determined by flow cytometry. We found that RSV binds to resting EOSs as well as those activated by platelet-activating factor (PAF) using a direct immunofluorescence method. Although RSV did not induce O_2^- generation by resting EOSs, RSV enhanced O_2^- generation of EOSs primed with PAF. Enhancement was significantly inhibited by either continuous agitation to prevent EOS adhesion to test tube surfaces or by pretreating cells with anti-CD18 antibody, suggesting that the stimulatory effects of RSV on EOSs depend on cell adhesion via β2-integrins. Futhermore, RSV enhanced PAF-induced CD11b expression by EOSs. These findings indicate that RSV enhances EOS CD11b expression and O_2^- generation induced by PAF. Thus, RSV infection may exacerbate airway inflammation by enhancing mediator release from human EOSs.

Role of Prostanglandin D_2 in the Pathogenesis of Bronchial Asthma

Kyoko Honda[a], Masafumi Arima[a,b], Gang Cheng[a], Fukiko Eda[a], Hirokuni Hirata[a], Fumiya Fukushima[a], Takeshi Fukuda[a]

[a]Department of Pulmonary Medicine and Clinical Immunology, Dokkyo University School of Medicine, Dokkyo, [b]Department of Developmental Genetics, Chiba University Graduate School of Medicine, Chiba, Japan

The pathogenesis of bronchial asthma is now well recognized as a persistent allergic inflammation. Prostaglandin D_2 (PGD_2), a major lipid mediator, is released from mast cells, but little is known about its role in the development of allergic reactions. Recently, PGD_2 signaling has been shown to regulate asthmatic inflammation via Th2-type response. We endeavored to clarify the role of PGD_2 in the airway inflammation of asthma. BALB/c mice were intraperitoneally sensitized with alum-absorbed OVA (8 μg) on days 0 and 5. On day 16, the mice were administered nebulized PGD_2 (10 μM) or saline as control for 30 min prior to challenge with aerosolized OVA (1 mg/ml sterile saline) for 30 min on day 17. The concentration of OVA was preliminarily established as causing a faint airway inflammation. We analyzed these mice 24 h post-OVA challenge. The numbers of eosinophils (EOSs) and lymphocytes in the bronchoalveolar lavage (BAL) fluid were significantly greater in PGD_2-pretreated mice than in control mice. Furthermore, PGD_2-pretreated mice showed an increased in airway hypersensitivity to inhaled methacholine, which was not observed in control mice. The levels of IL-4 and IL-5 in BAL fluid were also significantly higher in PGD_2-pretreated mice than in control mice, while the level of IFN-γ in the BAL fluid was not detectable in both mice. However, PGD_2 (0.1–100 μM) did not influence the cytokine production by antigen-stimulated splenic cells from intraperitoneally sensitized mice in vitro. In histological study, greater expression of macrophage-derived chemokaine (MDC), a chemoattractant for Th2 cells was observed in PGD_2-pretreated mice than that in control mice. Finally, intravenous administration of anti-MDC antibody into PGD_2-pretreated mice dramatically inhibited airway inflammation, Th2 cytokine production, and airway hypersensitivity after antigen challenge. Thus, PGD_2 caused an increase in the levels of Th2 cytokines and a chemokine, accompanied by the enhanced accumulation of EOSs and lymphocytes in the lung. A part of the PGD_2-evoked Th2 type inflammation might be contributed by MDC-induced recruitment of Th2 cells in the lung. These results indicate that PGD_2 plays an important role in the pathogenesis of chronic bronchial asthma with persistence of Th2 type inflammation.

Effect of Cetirizine on the Production of Reactive Oxygen Species from Human Eosinophils

Yoshiyuki Yamada, Satoshi Sannohe, Norihiro Saito, Chang-Hao Cui, Shigeharu Ueki, Hajime Oyamada, Akira Kanda, Kazutoshi Yamaguchi, Tetsuya Adachi, Hiroyuki Kayaba, Junichi Chihara

Department of Clinical and Laboratory Medicine, Akita University School of Medicine, Akita, Japan

Eosinophils play an important role in the development of allergic diseases such as asthma. Once migrated in the tissue, the cells release cytotoxic products including granule proteins and reactive oxygen species (ROS) leading to epithelial damage. We have previously shown that eotaxin possesses a priming effect on ROS production from eosinophils. Although cetirizine is effective in attenuating allergic inflammation, little is known about its direct action on eosinophils. In the present study, we studied the effect of cetirizine on eotaxin-primed ROS production from eosinophils. Eosinophils were isolated from peripheral blood in subjects with slight eosinophilia by a modified CD16– depletion method. After pretreatment with or without cetirizine, eosinophils were primed by eotaxin for 15 min followed by stimulation with calcium ionophore A23187. The production of ROS was measured by luminol-dependent chemiluminescence. Cetirizine had no effect on the production of ROS from eosinophils in the absence of eotaxin. In contrast, the ROS production from eotaxin-primed eosinophils was dose-dependently reduced by cetirizine (0.01–1 μg/ml). We demonstrated that cetirizine selectively suppressed the oxidative metabolism in eosinophils. It is possible that new-generation H_1-blockers such as cetirizine are a strategy for the treatment of allergic diseases through their direct effect on eosinophils.

Different Response to Chemokines in Reactive Oxygen Species Production from Eosinophils

Satoshi Sannohe[a,b], Yoshiyuki Yamada[a], Norihiro Saito[a], Chang-hao Cui[a], Tetsuya Adachi[a], Hiroyuki Kayaba[a], Kazuo Ishikawa[b], Junichi Chihara[a]

Departments of [a]Clinical and Laboratory Medicine and [b]Otolaryngology, Akita University School of Medicine, Akita, Japan

It has been shown that eosinophils from normal subjects and allergic patients were not functionally equivalent. The latter exhibit upregulated functions, such as chemotactic response and mediator release. In this study, we examined the functional characteristics of eosinophils in chemokine-primed production of reactive oxygen species (ROS).

After pretreatment with chemokines, eosinophils were stimulated with Ca ionophore A23187. ROS production from eosinophils was measured by luminol-dependent chemiluminescence.

Both RANTES and eotaxin possessed a priming effect on Ca-ionophore-induced ROS production from eosinophils. This effect was significantly enhanced in eosinophils from the patients. IL-5 was additionally augmentative for the priming effect of chemokines in eosinophils from normal subjects, but not from allergic subjects.

We demonstrated an enhanced response to chemokines in eosinophils from allergic patients. Our results suggest that IL-5 is involved in this enhancement.

International Archives of
Allergy and
Immunology

Int Arch Allergy Immunol 2002;128(suppl 1):28

List of Lectures by Speakers Who Have Not Submitted Their Manuscripts

Regulation of Ecalectin/Galectin-9 Production and Release in T Lymphocytes

Yumiko Kashio et al.
Department of Immunology and Immunopathology, Kagawa Medical School, Kagawa, Japan

Galectin-9 Expression in a Human Fibroblast Cell Line, HFL-1

Hirofumi Asakura et al.
Department of Radiology, Kagawa Medical School, Kagawa, Japan

Expression of Galectin-9 in an Experimental Asthmatic Model of Guinea Pigs

Hitomi Yamamoto et al.
Department of Pharmacology, Kyoto Pharmaceutical University, Kyoto, Japan

Human Mast Cells Induced Eosinophil Adhesion to Endothelial Cells in vitro

Motohiro Ebisawa et al.
Division of Pediatric Allergy, National Sagamihara Hospital Clinical Research Center, Kanagawa, Japan

Role of Eosinophil-Active Cytokines in Eosinophil Migration through Activated Epithelial Cells

Toshio Shimizu et al.
Department of Pediatric Allergy, Saku Central Hospital, Nagano, Japan

Expression of Fucosyltransferase-IV and -VII mRNA in Eosinophils

Takahiro Satoh et al.
Department of Dermatology and Immunodermatology, Graduate School, Tokyo Medical and Dental University, Tokyo, Japan

Transcription Factors Binding to the Promoter Region of the Murine IL-5 Receptor α Subunit Gene

Yuki Ashizawa et al.
Division of Immunology, Department of Microbiology and Immunology, Institute of Medical Science, University of Tokyo, Tokyo, Japan

Analysis of IL-5-Induced ERK Activation Pathway in Human Eosinophils

Masaki Hiraguri et al.
Department of Internal Medicine II, Chiba University School of Medicine, Chiba, Japan

Matrix Metalloproteinase-9 Release from Human Leukocytes

Shigeru Takafuji et al.
Department of Internal Medicine, St. Marianna University School of Medicine, Kawasaki, Japan

Gene Expression Analysis in Human Peripheral Blood Eosinophils by Various Cytokine Stimuli

Ryoichi Hashida et al.
Genox Research Inc. Kawasaki Lab., Kawasaki, Japan

The Relationship between Eosinophil Necrosis and ECP Value in Nasal Secretin

Tomonori Eguchi et al.
Department of Otolaryngology, Koshigaya Hospital, Dokkyo University School of Medicine, Saitama, Japan

KARGER

Fax + 41 61 306 12 34
E-Mail karger@karger.ch
www.karger.com

© 2002 S. Karger AG, Basel

Accessible online at:
www.karger.com/journals/iaa